Choosing Who's to Live

Ethics and Aging

Edited by
James W. Walters

University of Illinois Press
Urbana and Chicago

© 1996 by the Board of Trustees of the University of Illinois
Manufactured in the United States of America
1 2 3 4 5 C P 5 4 3 2 1
This book is printed on acid-free paper.
Library of Congress Cataloging-in-Publication Data
Choosing who's to live : ethics and aging / edited by James W.
  Walters.
     p.   cm.
Includes bibliographical references and index.
ISBN 0-252-02240-8 (cloth : acid-free paper). —
ISBN 0-252-06541-7 (pbk. : acid-free paper)
1. Aged—Medical care—Moral and ethical aspects. 2. Health care
rationing. 3. Aged—Medical care—Economic aspects. I. Walters,
James W. (James William), 1945–   .
RA564.8.C465   1996
174'.24—dc20   95-41785
                                                     CIP

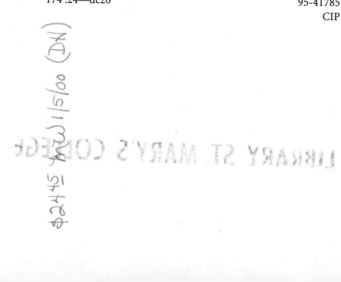

Contents

Acknowledgments

The essays in this volume evolved from a working conference held at Loma Linda University in 1991 that was designed to further the discussion of rationing health care beyond a focus on age as the primary criterion. The conference was part of a year-long Ethics and Aging Project, funded by the National Endowment for the Humanities. Special gratitude is expressed to David Larson, codirector of LLU's Ethics Center, who played a key role in conceptualizing the conference and this book's organization. Graduate students Duane Covrig and Brian Brock, as well as faculty secretary Gayle Foster, were invaluable in helping to bring these essays to publishable form.

Introduction

James W. Walters

Bill Clinton made health care reform a central feature of his 1992 presidential campaign, promising universal care and stabilized medical costs. What no one seemed to notice amidst all the political hoopla was that these two things are mutually exclusive without some sort of rationing.

Average Americans rebel at the thought of any kind of medical rationing, seeing unlimited health care on demand as one of our "inalienable rights." But we have to face the fact that *de facto* rationing is occurring already as a function of economic necessity and will grow in practice in a disorganized fashion unless we bring some reasoned management to bear on it. The outcome will not necessarily be disastrous. Canada spends far less of its gross domestic product on health care, yet maintains superior statistics on key indicators such as infant mortality and life expectancy. They do this by rationing health care.

Beyond the need to control costs and cover all citizens, there are at least four compelling arguments for facing the issue of rationing now:

1. The number of U.S. citizens over age eighty-five will increase 500 percent by 2040.
2. Current baby boomers could outlive today's elderly by seven to fifteen years.
3. New, increasingly expensive medical technologies come to market each year.
4. The tax base is shrinking. In forty years, the ratio of workers to retirees will be 1:4 instead of the current 1:2.5.

The first serious debate on health care rationing was sparked by the publication of *Setting Limits: Medical Goals in an Aging Society* (Simon and Schuster, 1987), by Daniel Callahan, philosopher and director of the Hastings Center, a center for ethical studies in the state of New York. Callahan called for mandatory age-based rationing of medical care, wherein patients eighty years old and older would be considered to have lived a "natural life span" and would be asked to accept "a tolerable death." Response to Callahan's thesis from the bioethics community has been largely negative.[1]

In this book six scholars representing bioethics, sociology, philosophy, and religious studies take this crucial debate beyond Callahan into the next round of discussion. In the first section, philosophers Paul Menzel and Norman Daniels outline their versions of what a prudent citizen would desire and expect in terms of lifetime health care. In the second section, philosopher Margaret Battin and bioethicist Nancy Jecker consider rationing in terms of euthanasia and long-term care. The final section of the book includes a critical analysis of bioethics by a team of medical sociologists from the University of California, San Francisco, and a humanistic reflection on ethics and aging by religious studies specialist John Kilner.

Unlike Callahan, who proposes a communitarian ethic in which elderly patients are asked to sacrifice for the greater good of society, Menzel and Daniels offer a less ethically stringent, more attainable agenda based on prudence.

Daniels further develops and refines his Prudential Lifespan Account as a conceptual approach to rationing medical resources. In this model, prudent persons would imagine themselves living beyond their current needs, and allocate scarce health care resources for each stage of their lives. In practice, this means that over the course of their lives, people would be treated justly, if quite differently. For instance, Daniels argues, it is prudent and morally just that the young should consume a disproportionate amount of resources, that wage earners should pay a disproportionate amount of taxes, and that the elderly should receive a disproportionate share of subsidized health care. Looking at the big picture, all get their fair share.

Daniels's Prudential Lifespan Account is not age-based, at least in principle. He sees the current focus on rationing health care according to age as "diversionary." He would rather we focus on when it is appropriate to give priority to the seriously ill and when it is not.

Menzel borrowed from some of Daniels's earlier work in developing his Prudent Consent model, which, he argues, incorporates the moral principle of integrity while avoiding the pitfall of free-riding. Integrity, according to Menzel, is a willing commitment to a rational allocation of health resources over a lifetime. Free-riding is taking advantage of a health care system funded by all citizens for their mutual benefit.

Like Daniels, Menzel argues that his prudential approach to rationing is not age-based, but "age-influenced," or, more accurately, life-expectancy and life-quality influenced. He believes that prudent consumers would reject grossly disproportionate health care in their final years if it meant extending low-quality life at great cost. He vigorously denies that the elderly would have lifesaving care withheld because they are "less deserving," for if they were living according to his Prudent Consent model, they would have given prior consent to less aggressive care in certain circumstances.

In the second section of this book, two philosophers grapple with the principle of self-determination for the elderly, and end up going in quite different directions. Margaret Battin makes a case for legalizing voluntary, active euthanasia; Nancy Jecker argues for transferring significant funds from acute to long-term health care.

To the question, "Is there a place for euthanasia in America's care for its elderly?" Battin answers "yes," if the model is the voluntary euthanasia practiced in the Netherlands. Shift the model to Nazi Germany, and her answer is an unequivocal "no."

Battin argues that the fundamental difference between these two models has created a lot of confusion in America over euthanasia. For the Dutch, self-determination is the key to ethical euthanasia. In Nazi Germany, of course, euthanasia was a system of killing people against their wills. While self-determination is Battin's guiding principle for accepting euthanasia, she does acknowledge an economic side to the argument for euthanizing terminally ill patients.

Jecker, on the other hand, argues that for millions of Americans the very idea of self-determination is being compromised by our egregious neglect of long-term care. Self-determination and self-respect are undermined when the elderly can no longer take care of their own basic needs. We consign them to a status of unequal worth and dignity when we deny them the opportunity to bathe, toilet, dress, and move about independently.

Currently, 50 percent of long-term care is paid out-of-pocket by those who need it; only 10 percent is paid for directly by those needing acute care. Jecker believes that the growing class of elderly citizens will cede more and more self-determination unless the government shifts health resources from acute to long-term care.[2]

In the last section, sociologist Carroll Estes and two associates, Elizabeth Binney and Susan Kelly, critique the discipline of bioethics on its assessment of ethics and aging. And finally, bioethicist John Kilner reflects on age-based rationing from a broadly humanistic perspective.

In her earlier work, Estes has lamented the "medicalization" of society's care for the elderly. Here, she and her team of authors criticize bioethics for adopting a narrow vision of human health. Just as modern doctors have focused on the "micro," individualistic aspects of their profession, opting for "medical care" instead of "health care," so bioethicists have idealized the individual, taking freely made contracts between rational individuals as the model for ethical relations. This emphasis on the needs of the individual is certainly in sync with American tradition and culture, but it removes the individual from any religious, social, cultural, or historical context and robs bioethics of a necessary communitarian perspective.

Estes and her colleagues challenge bioethicists to adopt a more critical approach to health care, one that recognizes the social, political, and economic issues inherent in the debate and includes gender, race, and class in the discussion of health care rationing. This broader perspective will take bioethicists beyond a high-tech medical agenda, to grapple with the broader issues of public health, preventive care, and chronic and long-term care. As Estes et al. see it, latching onto age as the basis for a solution to the health care crisis oversimplifies a highly complex issue.

The book's final chapter, by John Kilner, places the current interest in age-based rationing in the broader contexts of economics, politics, religion, and society. He criticizes our culture for its utilitarian approach to health care—maximizing pleasure for the great number of younger citizens at the expense of adequate care for the vulnerable elderly. Our society's interest in a "quick fix" has weakened our veneration for the old and led to an acceptance of voluntary active euthanasia as an answer to the health care crisis. Kilner is alarmed at this trend toward devaluing the elderly. That a society which spends $3 billion a year on potato chips would spawn a serious discussion of curtailing lifesaving treatment of the old as a way to conserve medical resources is understandable, he feels, but not right.

Notes

1. See Paul Homer and Martha Holstein, eds., *A Good Old Age?* (New York: Simon and Schuster, 1990); and Robert L. Barry and Gerard C. Bradley, eds., *Set No Limits: A Rebuttal to Daniel Callahan's Proposal to Limit Health Care for the Elderly* (Urbana: University of Illinois Press, 1991).

2. Jecker also points out the disproportionate burden elder care places on women. First, women far outlive men, and second, 75 percent of unpaid caregivers to the elderly are women.

Part 1
Justifications

1

The Justification and Implications of Age-Influenced Rationing

Paul T. Menzel

Three Types of Justification

One breakdown of the moral justifications of rationing health care would divide them into three sorts.

We can ground rationing in notions of distributive justice and the rights of individuals in a just society. Until all persons receive a certain basic level of care, for example, we might think that others have no right to be provided care that is significantly less basic. Let me call this simply the "Justice" justification of rationing. Here I would place the views of Robert Veatch and (sometimes) Norman Daniels.[1]

Alternatively, we can base rationing not primarily on the notion of a just society and the rights and deserts of individuals therein, but on ideals for the connectedness and solidarity of a community of persons. In relation to age-based rationing in particular, justifications in this category might urge the revision of our cultural conception of aging to allow the elderly to live more meaningful lives as members of a consciously intergenerational community. Daniel Callahan, for example, urges precisely this: the elderly gain a new meaning for their lives by passing the torch of life on to subsequent generations.[2] Let me call this the "Communitarian Ideal" justification of age-based rationing: it aims to connect the elderly individual to the larger intergenerational community, and it aspires to promote a conception of the meaning of old age that is currently probably not widely shared (at least not widely shared in a strong enough form to generate a basis for rationing).

A third type of justification for rationing works from people's prudential (rational and self-interested) choices about how to allocate the scarce resources among the multiple needs and goals of their lives. This I call the "Prudent Consent" justification for rationing. In this category can be found Daniels's view in his book on distributing health care between young and old, and my own work both on rationing in general and age-related rationing in particular.[3]

In this chapter I only want to make two brief comments about the Justice and Communitarian Ideal justifications for rationing health care before I move on to more detailed observations about Prudent Consent. These comments are perhaps crude and hasty generalizations, but let me make them quickly nonetheless.

First, the Justice and Communitarian Ideal justifications start with a certain conception about the nature of the primary moral problem in rationing: we face a dilemma between meeting the needs of the individual patient (to whom health care providers, at least, have traditionally been presumed to be loyal) and attending to certain societal needs—for Justice models, a just pattern of relationships among persons, and for Communitarian Ideal models, the welfare of a society with cohesive culture that gives meaning to the lives of individuals. Proponents of these models are inclined to think that a fundamentally new ethic is now needed for health care delivery. Either attention to patient needs will have to be subordinated to qualifications of just distribution involving the whole society, or the individual centered values of patient welfare and autonomy will have to take second place to considerations of achieving a more constructive place for the patient in the intergenerational community. If this is correct, a fundamental shift away from thinking in terms of individual prudence or consent will be necessary for people to accept rationing as morally defensible. In the larger moral-cultural context, then, rationing will require a certain crucial amount of "moral missionary" work: getting people to give up their attachment to their own individual goals and interests and acknowledge a larger justice or social cohesiveness. I am not strictly opposed to embarking on such an effort; I only want to note that it is a very tall order indeed, especially in an American culture that has emphasized the primacy of individuals and their attendant rights and freedoms.

Second, it is difficult to get much consensus on either the substantive content of justice or on the claim that the primary meaning of our old age resides in passing the torch of life on to the young. The Justice model does not shrink from finally imposing just policies on recalcitrant individuals, but we first have to come to a modicum of agreement in the society on what constitutes justice. Advocates of the Communitarian Ideal like Callahan, on the other hand, hesitate to impose their ideal on others, but what, realistically, is the likelihood that enough people will voluntarily start thinking in roughly their way to generate policies and widespread social practices rather than merely constituting an interesting (even noticeable) segment of society?

By contrast, the likelihood of Prudent Consent justifications getting widely acknowledged as legitimate grounds for denying an individual patient beneficial care is greater. The moral ground such justifications plow is already part of American culture. Prudent Consent justifications of rationing start by inquiring into people's own judgments about the policies they would want to determine their health care, considering all the realities of cost and scarcity. If individual patients would prudently consent to substantive and procedural policies of restricting certain care, the appeal of those policies will rest not merely on attachment to the morally controversial goal of increasing aggregate societal welfare or serving some particular, probably disputed pattern of justice, but on respect for patients' own will and long-term self-interest.

One way to sum up the whole (and limited) point of the Prudent Consent model is to see it as simply a straightforward response to the two most common objections to rationing: (1) it is said that citizens of the United States, at least, will not tolerate the rationing out of their own possible care; they want everything, and the best, for their own case; (2) providers object to rationing as a violation of their fidelity to patients. The Prudent Consent model meets the first objection head-on by claiming that some rationing out of possibly beneficial care is what people do want; if they consider their own realities of cost and scarcity, they will not endorse policies, public or private, that provide everything in their own future case. Prudent Consent meets the second objection by explaining how providers' participation in rationing can respect both the best interest and autonomy of patients; by not participating in subscriber-patient endorsed rationing, in fact, providers are violating their fidelity to patients.[4]

An Example, and a Clarification about Terminology

To clarify the essential structure of Prudent Consent justifications of age-related rationing, consider the following choice.[5]

You are thirty. You can purchase coverage for any of three treatments for five dollars per month each, paid from age thirty to sixty-five (whether you ever need the treatment or not):

Treatment A: for disease generally striking at age 30–50.
Treatment B: for disease generally striking at age 50–70.
Treatment C: for disease generally striking over age 70.

If your likelihoods of needing A, B, and C are equal, would you not buy coverage first for A, then for B, and lastly for C? Furthermore, will you not verify the prudential justification of that priority ranking even when you are seventy? Keep in mind in this conceptual scenario just what you are being asked to reflect on at seventy: you are being asked to endorse a policy *for your lifetime,* not just express what you might want now for the rest of your life.

To be sure, just as someone at seventy could refuse to take seriously the real question of allocation that is at issue (a choice for a lifetime), so also someone at thirty could refuse to consider seriously any part of their likely life over fifty (or seventy, or whatever). Indeed, we should regard the refusal of a thirty-year-old to invest in any policy that provides life-prolonging care after seventy as irrational. If the care eliminated were exceedingly inexpensive, high benefit care ($50 to save a life, for example), and one were already gladly spending at the rate of $50,000 or $500,000 per life saved at younger ages, why wouldn't one shift a tiny bit of the resources at the top margin of that latter investment so that one could handle very cheap-to-save situations in satisfactory quality-of-life old age?

The answers that prudent individuals are likely to give to such questions reveal that what prudence in fact endorses is not any real *age*-rationing at all. In making prudential choices to shape our future, we will not endorse any age-line cut-off for life extending care. Age only influences our earlier prudent investment choice in two respects, and then only indirectly, not as a matter of age per se. Age will influence prudent choice to the extent that an investment in care delivered in old age is likely to save a much shorter span of life than equally likely-to-save-life care will save at a younger age, and it will influence it to the extent that we estimate the quality of the life that will be saved in old age to be low. It is even misleading to call this kind of influence and its results age-*based* rationing, for it is neither *based on* age, nor is it even *directly* influenced by age. It is only rationing *indirectly influenced by* a characteristic of age—that other things being equal (and sometimes they are not!), one has less life yet to live if one is saved in old age than one has left when one is saved at a younger age.[6] The rationing that is justified by Prudent Consent is thus only indirectly age-influenced.

Moral Backbone and the Implementation of Prudent Consent

We have previously seen that Prudent Consent requires less in the way of controversial moral claims than Justice and Communitarian Ideal models do. Both in its conclusions concerning age and in its necessary moral assumptions, Prudent Consent, compared to Justice, is morally a lowest common denominator approach to rationing, and it is certainly a lower common denominator approach than any Communitarian Ideal justification could possibly be at the present stage of our cultural history. At the same time, however, it is worth noting that some very substantive moral principles and ideals are at work in the Prudent Consent model. I call the more obvious one Integrity, and I refer to the other as Avoidance of Free-Riding.

Integrity

Assume it is prudent for each of the members of a group to endorse restricting lifesaving care in old age more than care at a younger age when both are nominally equally expensive because the care in the older-age case has a significantly lower benefit-cost ratio. Why should people finally implement such prudent restrictions on care for elderly patients who at the time might still benefit from it immensely? A sufficient answer must say something more about the need to make judgments about, and implement policies for, extensive spans of life.

Given the insurance-centered structure of a modern health care economy, controlling the use of even very high-cost-per-benefit care is extremely difficult. Once patients are insured, whether in private or in public arrangements, both they and providers have strong incentives to use care even when its statistical benefits approach zero and its cost is still high. To respond to this problem and regain some control over insurance-supported medicine's otherwise virtually endless draw on resources, subscribers and patients must see resource use from a longer temporal vantage point than simply that of a vulnerable and hurting patient. Equally, of course, it should not be the perspective of an earlier subscriber who fails to imagine realistically what it is to be ill. But in any case, it should certainly not be a person now seen only as a temporally limited "patient." Knowing what incentives are created by insurance, the problem of controlling the use of care has to be addressed, in our *conceptual* thinking, at least, at an early point in the process. After all, such a point, insuring, is where the essential trouble starts.

My claim about integrity here is essentially simple: patients and subscribers of integrity will not shrink from this task of addressing the explosion of health care resource use at a point in time prior to being the actual patient who could use the care. Integrity is *the managing of one's life, and the resources for one's life, over time.* In their later situation as insured and ill patients, people's realistic capacity to control the resources of their larger lives is sharply diminished. Whether in communities or as individuals, it is the potential for integrity that allows us to retrieve control.

It seems correct, even obviously correct, to say all this about subscribers, taxpayers, and voters in reference to a fairly limited span of time, say the one-year period for which they enroll in a health plan. The point would also seem to hold, however, for longer time-spans of our lives. A significant source of the escalation of health care costs is that we are increasingly becoming a statistically older population. That, combined with the fact that the real cost per statistical unit of benefit for many specific items of care in old age can be unusually high, means that the cost of health care for the aged is a major problem for our lives as a whole. Why would integrity limit its scope to the relatively short spans of life for which one insures with an annual premium? The *ideal* of integrity, at least, asks us to take account of our long-range needs in the context of what we want our lives to be as a whole.

Avoidance of Free-Riding

Closely related to the moral demands of integrity in Prudent Consent's generation of health care rationing are moral requirements to avoid free-riding. To set the stage here, let me back up, state more precisely a principle about free-riding, and set the larger context for its use in health care policy to restrict patients' and providers' range of action.

One famous argument, the argument from "public goods" and free-riding, has often been thought to provide a genuine reconciliation of a state's or group's coercive power with individual liberty: if the essential benefits of collective policies accrue to everyone—the goods are "public" and "nonexclusive"[7]—a group may extract from all individuals their fair share of the costs of those policies (obedience, say, or taxes). Otherwise the recalcitrant noncontributors are "free-riding": obtaining the benefits without paying their proportionate cost. In terms of respecting the individual, the nice thing about such an argument for the collective's right to enforce policies is that behind it still lies the fact of *the individual's preference* for the collective policies.

What I call the Anti-Free-Riding Principle (AFRP) that drives this argument can be stated more precisely.[8] Regarding receipt of benefits, AFRP holds that: No person should receive nonexclusive benefits from a collective enterprise without paying their fair share of its costs, as long as they would be willing to pay that share rather than lose all benefits of the enterprise entirely.[9]

I have argued elsewhere that the correct limiting condition in this part of the principle is precisely the benefit-receiving person's hypothetical consent conveyed in the statement above.[10] It is not the weaker condition of a person's mere "acceptance" of the benefits, and unless consulting people for their actual prior consent is feasible and not prohibitively costly, it is not the stronger condition of their actual consent. If in fact people really *would* have agreed to pay their share rather than forego the benefits, and if the context is already stipulated as one where we are dealing with the kind of good from which it is very difficult if not impossible to exclude noncontributors, then it is entirely respectful of people as free individuals to hold them responsible for contributing their share.[11] (I will return to this point in the next section on presumptions of prudent consent.)

Put this now in the context of rationing health care. If better alternate use of resources is the good that persons in a private or public insurance pool receive by constraining the use of high-cost/low-benefit care, anyone desiring to receive that benefit must pay their fair share of the costs necessary to produce it. In the case of rationing health care, this share is simply abiding by limitations on care when they are applied to one's own later case as a patient. Not to abide by these restrictions, when they are indeed necessary to achieve the benefit, is free-riding if the context is one where others largely do abide by them. Noncontributors would be receiving the common benefit of lower premiums or taxes without shouldering their own share of the burdens. (Physicians who would deliver services to their patients that lie outside the limitations that pre-patient members of the pool think represent the best use of resources would also be free-riding. They fail to do their necessary part in the collective rationing enterprise, while they still receive the general benefit of belonging to a profession that consumers or citizens now regard as delivering only cost-worthy services instead of breaking the bank.)

Of course, any argument that people must pay their share is only as good as the descriptive accuracy of the claim that they have in fact agreed, or would have agreed, to pay their share to get the benefits. I will pursue the interesting questions that surround making such a claim in the next section on presumptions of prudent consent. For now, note only that the avoidance of free-riding, though it is a moral good, is itself a fundamentally individualist value that does not require resort to ambitious calls to reform American morality along more just or communitarian lines. In holding people responsible not merely for the effects of their voluntary actions on others but also for the costs of the collective enterprises from which they benefit, the Anti-Free-Riding Principle keeps collective solutions to human needs in tow, tying them more tightly than they would otherwise be to people's ability and willingness to pay their costs. The moral need to avoid free-riding provides constructive connection between social arrangements and individual responsibility.

Implementing the rationing policies generated by Prudent Consent thus requires strong moral values of its own: integrity, the responsibility to manage one's life and the resources for it over time, and the obligation not to free-ride but to pay one's fair share of the costs of collective policies that it is prudent for one to endorse. Prudence can at first look like a morally uninspiring call to arms in the move toward rationing health care responsibly in our society. In fact it presupposes strong ideals and values of its own, though it has the advantage of not demanding a major shift in the underlying moral culture of the United States.

It is possible, of course, that the values of integrity and the avoidance of free-riding are already so weak in American culture that Prudent Consent will require a tremendous amount of "moral missionary" work of its own. I do not necessarily deny that, but I would still note one important point: integrity and the avoidance of free-riding are values that people more broadly and less controversially pay at least lip service to than they do to any further substantive principle of justice or strong ideal of intergenerational solidarity. For Prudent Consent, the moral call that is undoubtedly required for any approach to rationing health care to gain public acceptance can be made on the basis of traditional values that the culture already claims.

Presumptions of Prudent Consent, and the Case of Helga Wanglie

We can rather easily justify the claim that if push comes to shove in the competition of different goals for the limited resources available for a lifetime, one would be prudent to consider the relatively short lengths of life typically added by lifesaving care in old age. The truth of that claim does not by itself generate a sufficient justification for restricting selective lifesaving services for the elderly, however. If the prudence of such policies is our focus, we will have to face accusations of parentalistically overriding the expectations that competent individuals have for their care (that it will not be rationed when they are ill and vulnerable). If, on the other hand, the consent prong of Prudent Consent arguments is thought to carry the primary burden of moral justification, we must heed the fact that few people actually consent to limitations on their care. For one thing, people seldom even think of themselves as making allocation choices for later stages of life. It is rarer yet for people in our society to make any explicit, age-influenced rationing decision like deleting Treatment C from coverage. Furthermore, many of the explicit advance decisions that people could readily make are crude: to delete an entire type of treatment from coverage, say, without distinguishing what may be the greatly different cost-benefit characteristics of that treatment in different individual clinical circumstances. What Prudent Consent justifications of rationing will often actually have to rely on, then, are presumptions about hypothetical prudent consent: what actual patient-subscribers would previously have prudently consented to delete had they considered the sort of situation in which they now happen to find themselves.

What moral weight, however, does merely presumed, hypothetical consent carry? Ideally, of course, subscribers or their representatives should be actively involved in actually shaping the major priorities and guidelines in rationing services to increase cost worthiness. For one thing, people see intrinsic value in making their own explicit choices. But, as I have argued elsewhere, this is not consent's sole value.[12] Bringing decisions in line with a person's values and beliefs is also a major component in the moral importance of what we speak of as "consent." To test this out, consider some examples where the only consent possible is hypothetical and presumed. Suppose you are comatose. Should we simply say that since there is obviously no intrinsic value any longer in your now impossible explicit participation, we are going to make the decision about whether to keep you alive solely on the basis of *our* values? Both in relation to any future you may have if you ever wake up, and in relation to the value you already have had in living a life and approaching a death that is your own, it is important that we conceptually consult what you would decide were you conscious.[13]

The moral legitimacy of presuming the hypothetical consent of actual persons, though, is contingent on several crucial conditions. First, there must be sufficient reason for referring back to a temporally earlier consent rather than just leaving the matter to later, unconstrained decision.[14] Second, it must have been either impossible or prohibitively costly to have actually consulted people about whether they would agree to restrict later care.[15] Without these two conditions we should have to put up or shut up about consent—either look again for actual consultation and consent or forego use of any claims about what the person would have prudently decided. In fact, however, in health care rationing contexts, these two essential conditions are frequently (though not always) present.[16]

Moreover, the moral weight of accurately hypothesized prudent consent is considerably bolstered or weakened by two other circumstantial factors. The more clearly and explicitly the entire context of care and its coverage is lean delivery and acknowledgment of concern for efficiency, the more ethical room there is for presuming a person's consent to rationing out marginal care. On the other hand, the more an insurer or provider publicly proclaims that cost is never any consideration in covering or not covering (prescribing or not prescribing) care, the less plausible it probably is to claim that someone who is now a patient would have consented to restrictions. Both factors are important, but only insofar as they make more credible or suspicious the claim that the persons who are now the patients would have consented to restrictions had they actually been consulted.

The widely discussed 1991 Minnesota case of Helga Wanglie provides an interesting illustration of how such circumstantial considerations complicate the presuming of consent.[17] Mrs. Wanglie had been in a coma since

June 1990; by January 1991 both physicians and her husband and children agreed she would never regain consciousness. Nonetheless her family wished that the life-sustaining ventilator and feeding tubes be continued. Her physicians argued that such care was medically futile and that they therefore had no obligation to prescribe the care even if the family wanted it for Helga. She had left no clear or written instructions on the matter, though her husband quoted her as saying that "only He who gives life may take it." He interpreted this statement to mean that she would want to be given respiratory and nutritional support even when permanently comatose. Despite the fact that the cost of her care from November 1990, when the dispute between the family and physicians began to emerge, until July 1991, when she died of an infection, exceeded $700,000, her insurance company publicly stated all along that cost should not be a factor in treatment decisions; it was willing to pay for her care until a court approved its removal.[18]

Several things are clear about this case. First, it did not really involve the medical futility that her physicians claimed. Her ventilator and tube feedings kept her alive during these months, and since (being comatose) she was not in pain, her family's claim that life was still of some value to her (or to them and thereby to her) could hardly be denied outright by physicians.[19] At the same time, however, I think it highly likely that *if*, before all this happened, Helga Wanglie had been consulted seriously about whether she was willing to devote enough of her accessible resources to insure that even admittedly *permanently comatose* patients would be kept alive *at the cost of $1 million per year of life saved*, she would have preferred that the resources be spent on other things. We must hypothetically query her beforehand as facing *that* resource question, not the much less revealing question of whether she saw some value in a comatose life. When her physicians pressed to remove life support, therefore, they should have portrayed removal as permissible rationing of beneficial care, not withdrawal of care that had no benefit for the patient.

An anomalous factor, though, disturbs this presumed consent argument for rationing out Mrs. Wanglie's ventilator. Mrs. Wanglie's insurance company had publicly committed itself to the general proposition that cost of care is no object. No doubt that commitment was foolish (not to say, perhaps, dishonest), but since the commitment was publicly made, aren't we obligated to honor it as the company's commitment to Mrs. Wanglie in particular?

It may seem so, but I doubt it. While such a commitment had short-term public relations value for the insurer, we can still say that it was probably out of line with Mrs. Wanglie's real values. She may have *liked* to think that cost was no object in care decisions, but *if she had really confronted the bald resource trade-off question,* I think it is highly probable she would have agreed not to insure for care costing *$1 million per year of comatose life.* Even with the insurance company's public commitment, then, our guess that Mrs. Wanglie would not have been willing beforehand to devote the additional resources to cover expensive care to support comatose life is the most reasonable one to make.

But of course that "retrospective prediction" carries no certainty. And are we not required, out of respect for Mrs. Wanglie's dignity as an individual capable of making choices for her life, to have asked her beforehand for her actual consent to a care-denying policy? *Ideally,* indeed, we should have, but the question in a policy context is whether we *must* consult her for her actual consent when we can predict with some degree of reliability what her response to the real resource trade-off question would have been. Even in the most open, free market competition, insurance companies would probably not put detailed layouts of every sort of care covered or excluded before potential subscribers. More importantly, the best way to initiate the open, public discussion about care for the comatose that will lead subscribers and insurers to come to much clearer prior agreements to ration care is to put the ball in the other court: begin the public practice of excluding such care, putting the burden on any minority of subscribers with opposite convictions to seek out their own separate coverage. For one thing, that would test out the integrity of any who claim that cost should be no object in their care. Ironically, insisting on actually obtaining consent before we can begin any rationing may be a relatively ineffective way of eliciting people's real choices!

I suspect that at this time in our history the same analysis is appropriate for certain age-influenced segments of rationing. Public payers, insurance companies, and providers should begin to allow the length and quality of life that can be saved to shape decisions to forego some of the lowest-benefit, highest-expense procedures for elderly patients. When that is done, however, it should be done publicly enough to allow people to pursue the option of investing more in their future care to avoid later rationing. We have a long road to go here, but institutions must have the courage to stimulate the process of public and subscriber discussion.

As such a beginning, many insurance companies should immediately adopt explicit, membership-announced policies of excluding coverage for life support care for permanently comatose patients. That care is not necessarily futile, but our best guess is that the vast majority of people do not regard the benefits it brings as sufficient to warrant its real cost. If for particular individuals this judgment is mistaken, they can purchase alternate insurance.[20] The shoe should start falling on the other foot: people should be forced to think about these investments by having the responsibility to "buy up," if that is what they wish, instead of providers and insurers having to carry the burden of demonstrating futility or proving that an individual would not have chosen to pay for the extra, disputed coverage.

Perceptual Relativity and the Real Cost of Lifesaving

Persons of integrity take seriously the task of distributing over their lifetimes the accessible resources that they and others produce. Economic resources are not just "available" somehow from some big pot of resources. They are produced by people, and it is largely only through some such production that they are available to anyone at all. We have to realize that given what we produce, we have so much, and only so much, to use in our lifetimes. But that has implications above and beyond whether we should provide health care procedures just considering their cost alone. The plain fact is that the longer we live without producing proportionately more, the further we will have to stretch those resources even just for normal costs of living.

One of the implications that I have drawn from this point in previous writings is that the real, total costs of some nominally inexpensive health care services are often much higher than people perceive.[21] In the case of penicillin to treat the pneumonia of a nursing home patient, for example, the real cost is more like $35,000 per year of life saved, not $50 total. The key items in this calculation are the cost of continued nursing home care and other (perhaps unrelated) medical care that will be incurred if the penicillin works, and the pension benefits that will similarly continue to be paid. The fact that pension benefits or nursing home expenses may seem at this stage of life to be routine "costs of living," not the costs of discretionary health care, provides no defense against incorporating them in our calculation of the costs of a particular lifesaving act. In competition with other things in life, added pension benefits as well as the nursing home expenses are real costs of living longer. We have to see it this way once we move into this business of trying to gain control over the resources of our lives. In fact, then, from the very perspective we already occupy simply by discussing the limiting of what we spend on health care, we are compelled to consider the pension benefits and nursing home expenses for added years of life as real costs of lifesaving care. Thus, in this situation penicillin should be seen as approaching the same candidate-for-rationing ballpark of debatably cost-worthy limits as kidney dialysis, the most expensive-per-likely-benefit transplants and open heart surgeries, and diagnostic tests of statistically small return. People of integrity, appreciating all the ages they might live into, will not hide their heads in the sand about the real costs of lifesaving in old age.

Even stating all this vigorously, however, I must admit a distinct problem in carrying through on the point within the Prudent Consent model for making rationing decisions. Recognizing these costs, should we really think through what the prudent consent of subscribers would presumably be and conclude by denying coverage for the lifesaving penicillin and the resulting nursing home expenses it creates? If people *did* take responsibility for coming to *informed, prudent* judgments about how to allocate their accessible resources over their lifetimes, I think there is little question but that they would regard that use of penicillin as a very real candidate for restriction. Yet unlike a ventilator or feeding tube for a comatose Helga Wanglie, or even a potentially much more human-welfare producing procedure like a bypass graft on an elderly patient likely to live another few years, we find the penicillin for the nursing home patient distinctly more difficult to deny. Even amidst the immediate crisis requiring the care, people can take somewhat to heart the costs of Helga Wanglie's ventilator or the bypass graft, integrating them into the broader pattern of resource use over whole lifetimes. Bringing in pension benefits and routine nursing home expenses for a conscious patient in the penicillin-for-pneumonia case seems much more difficult. By including "ordinary" costs of living in the cost picture, we feel we are coming dangerously close to resenting the simple continuation of the person's life.

In the last analysis, I suspect that we should give considerable weight to such "perceptual relativities" in the application of the Prudent Consent model for rationing. We are straining the claim that Prudent Consent reconciles rationing with fidelity to the individual patient if we construe subscriber-patients as much more rational in sizing up all these trade-offs than they would even *want* to be regarded as being if they were to discuss this very meta-policy puzzle. As we get more accomplished in exercising and expanding our integrity in thinking about resource use over whole lifetimes, I would guess that this resistance to seeing and acting on certain items as real costs will subside, but at the present stage of the moral-cultural history of health policy we should not presume more rational and prudent consent than people are realistically capable of absorbing.

On this general matter of the historical policy context in which we think through these issues, we could note another interesting fact about the current United States situation. We do not have a single-payer system, nor do people have their care in earning years and old age provided through the same integrated plan. Medicare for the elderly is separated off from the rest of our system; furthermore, it is largely funded by current workers' earnings, not via a trust fund where future recipients pay in during their earning years the bulk of the very dollars that will provide for their later care. Thus people are not encouraged to think early on about what is worth funding in their later years. The structure of the system encourages us to think about what is worth providing in the later years only then when we are old. Since that is when we have finished making most of our contributions to the funding (current workers foot most of the bill), we are not likely ever to feel squarely confronted with the real trade-offs between the health care resources used in different segments of our lives. This deficiency is made all the worse by some employers' policy of guaranteeing Medicare-supplement coverage for retired workers but not significantly (or at all) funding it during those workers' earning years.[22]

Moving the health care financing structure in either direction—more private and individual, or more public and unified—would probably encourage better consideration of the lifetime distribution of resources. On this count our current system is the worst of all worlds. Obviously a more individual lifetime fund arrangement would encourage more entire-lifetime thinking, but so would a unified single-payer system. In the latter, voters and legislators would have to confront the distribution of resources in the whole system. If representatives successfully vote to add more funding for health care for the elderly, they will likely increase the pressure to provide fewer services for another stage of life. Though an age-unified single-payer system allows less individual responsibility for distribution of resources over the full age range, a congressperson's perspective in funding a unified system would tend to see health care policy as an integrated collection of decisions for the entire range of life's stages.

Are Women Disadvantaged by Age-Influenced Rationing?

Nancy Jecker has pointed out that age-based rationing raises questions of gender discrimination because more women than men constitute the elderly population that such rationing would seem to adversely affect. Over the age of eighty-five, women outnumber men more than two to one; over sixty-five, three to two. Women at sixty-five are likely to live another eighteen years, men only another fourteen.[23]

Indeed, rationing health care directly *by* age would adversely affect significantly more women than men. If rationing is guided by prior Prudent Consent, however, it is only indirectly age-*influenced,* and the results for women are somewhat different. Men whom we save with some acute care procedure at a given age like sixty-five are likely to live fewer additional years than women of the same age. If they are prudently rationing care over their lifetimes before they reach old age, men would have reason to put a lower priority on acute lifesaving care at sixty-five than women would; statistically speaking, men simply have less to gain from it. If the rationing of care in old age is allowed to be sensitive to the likely length of life that it will save or improve, as it certainly would be in a Prudent Consent approach, then women, in fact, may find their care rationed out *less* frequently than men!

If, of course, we more crudely restricted care solely by entire procedure/symptom categories, allowing no variation by amount of statistically likely gain, then age-influenced rationing might be more disadvantageous to women than to men. Especially if men hold more influence on public policy making, they might set restrictions applying both to men and to women on the basis of what it was prudent largely only for them (men) to accept (more age-influenced rationing). Since Jecker argues that "resource-centered" rationing omitting coverage for specific procedures is not as objectionable as "person-centered" rationing that selects out categories of people, she is likely to have the resource-centered variety in mind. She is then correct (for that variety of rationing) in charging that any age-based deletion of selected procedures that is not directly related to prognosis and statistical benefit is likely to take a greater toll on women than men. Age-influenced rationing, however, is not likely to be primarily procedure/resource centered. In focusing not on categories of procedures per se, but on the amount of likely benefit relative to cost, age-influenced rationing may at times look "person-centered." It would not be correct, however, to characterize any such rationing of this merely age-*influenced* type as resting on the idea of some people being "less deserving due to the kinds of people they are." No one who is denied lifesaving care in the Prudent Consent model is regarded as "less deserving." It is only that they are likely to benefit less from a given margin of extra health care expenditure than people whose care is not restricted. If indeed there are grounds for them to consent prudently to such restrictions beforehand, the rationing hardly affronts them as being less "deserving." On the other hand, if there are no such grounds and they did not consent (or would not have), then on the Prudent Consent model the rationing is already not justified; we do not even reach the more refined criticisms concerning different gender impact.

Admittedly, age-influenced rationing *could* succumb to the temptation to discount incorrectly the quality and value of a given length of life in old age as lower than the value of similar life spans at younger ages. That would be age-bias indeed, but it is not a necessary or even likely development in Prudent Consent justified rationing. While a year of younger life may often be of higher quality, it is important that we not stereotype the value of life in old age as automatically low. In particular it is important not to regard the quality of elderly women's lives as low just because of some stereotype of elderly women.

We should permit the rationing of health care to be influenced by the smaller number of years of life that are typically at stake in health care for the elderly. There are dangers, to be sure, to which any such rationing opens the door. These dangers can be guarded against, and we should not allow their possibility to push us off track from the task of responsibly controlling the resources of our lives.

Notes

1. I place some of Daniels's work in this category, especially "Why Saying No to Patients in the United States Is So Hard," *New England Journal of Medicine* 314 (May 22, 1986): 1381–83, but also, though less clearly about rationing, *Just Health Care* (Cambridge: Cambridge University Press, 1985). I would also include here Troyen Brennan, *Just Doctoring: Medical Ethics in the Liberal State* (Berkeley: University of California Press, 1991).

For age-based rationing in particular, justifications that emphasize something like "the right to a minimal age first" fall into this "justice" category. Taking a whole-lifetime perspective on equality, these justifications ask rhetorically why the foremost condition of all the other good things in life, time in life, shouldn't be the first thing distributed equally among us. See Robert Veatch, "Justice and Valuing Lives," in Robert Veatch, ed., *Life Span: Values and Life-Extending Technologies* (New York: Harper and Row, 1979), 197–224, as well as his contribution in James Walters and Gerald Winslow, eds., *Facing Limits: Ethics and Health Care for the Elderly* (Boulder: Westview Press, 1993). For discussions of this sort of view, see John Harris, *The Value of Life: An Introduction to Medical Ethics* (London: Routledge and Kegan Paul, 1985), 99–101; and Paul T. Menzel, *Medical Costs, Moral Choices: A Philosophy of Health Care Economics in America* (New Haven: Yale University Press, 1983), 190–93.

2. Daniel Callahan, *Setting Limits: Medical Goals in an Aging Society* (New York: Simon and Schuster, 1987). On rationing in general, not age-related rationing in particular, I would somewhat more tentatively include in this category Larry Churchill, *Rationing Health Care in America: Perceptions and Principles of Justice* (Notre Dame: University of Notre Dame Press, 1987).

3. Norman Daniels, *Am I My Parents' Keeper? An Essay on Justice between the Young and the Old* (New York: Oxford University Press, 1988). The use of "justice" in the title does not place his view in this book in my first category, though in a sense his view bridges both the "justice" and "prudence" categories. The larger point he makes is that rationing on the basis of age can be made compatible with justice, but his argument for this is "the Prudential Lifespan Account." Admittedly, I should perhaps not put his view under any label involving consent, for it is prudence, not actual or presumable consent, that drives his argument. Also, he frames the question of prudence within conditions of background justice: he argues that rationing according to age criteria can be just if it is a prudent arrangement for individuals already living in a basically just society. Clearly in the hypothetical prudent-consent-to-rationing view is Ronald Dworkin, "Will Clinton's Plan Be Fair?" *New York Review of Books,* Jan. 13, 1994, 20–25. For my views on rationing in general, see Paul T. Menzel, *Strong Medicine: The Ethical Rationing of Health Care* (New York: Oxford University Press, 1990); for age-related rationing in particular, see pp. 196–201 therein and section 4 of "Counting the Costs of Lifesaving Interventions for the Elderly," in Walters and Winslow, eds., *Facing Limits,* 137–50.

4. See Paul T. Menzel, "Double Agency and the Ethics of Rationing Health Care: A Response to Marcia Angell," *Kennedy Institute of Ethics Journal* 3:3 (Summer 1993): 287–92.

5. This is exactly the example I used in Menzel, "Counting the Costs of Lifesaving Interventions."

6. This point is reinforced by some other priorities we would prudently endorse for our later health care as elderly patients. We will clearly not commit ourselves to doing without palliative or chronic care in even the oldest of age. We might discount the relative priority of lifesaving care for old age because of considerable differences in the amount of life we save, but we will hardly condemn ourselves to misery and lack of care for any period of time when we will be alive in any case, even if that time is very old age indeed. Long-term and palliative care stay as high priority as they are for younger years (assuming similar costs and benefits per year).

7. Public safety, national defense, or the education of a populace to support a modern economy, for example. Once a certain mass of contributors is in place, it is difficult if not impossible to exclude from the benefits of these enterprises an individual who chooses not to contribute to them.

8. Technically, AFRP speaks to two situations, one where people actively impose costs on others and the other where they receive benefits without paying their share of expense. The latter is more applicable in our context, so I will only pursue this part of the principle.

9. This second component of the larger AFRP is widely known in the philosophical literature as the "Principle of Fairness" or the "Duty of Fair Play." See H. L. A. Hart, "Are Their Any Natural Rights?" *Philosophical Review* 64 (1955): 185–98; Robert Nozick, *Anarchy, State, and Utopia* (New York: Basic Books, 1974), 93–95; A. John Simmons, "The Principle of Fair Play," *Philosophy and Public Affairs* 8 (Summer 1979): 307–37; Richard Arneson, "The Principle of Fairness and Free-Rider Problems," *Ethics* 92 (Apr. 1982): 616–33; George Klosko, "Presumptive Benefit, Fairness, and Political Obligation," *Philosophy and Public Affairs* 6 (Summer 1987): 241–59; and Mario Morelli, "The Fairness Principle," *Philosophy and Law Newsletter of the American Philosophical Association* 6 (Spring 1985): 2–4. Note that the "fair share" and "willing to pay" elements in my statement of the principle already include the exemption that would often be claimed for people unable to pay. In their case, either the fair share of payment is virtually nothing, or, with their meager resources they would not have been willing to pay to get the benefits; they thus have no duty to pay just because we cannot now exclude them from the benefits. On the general point about not obligating people unable to pay, see David Schmidtz, *The Limits of Government: An Essay on the Public Goods Argument* (Boulder: Westview Press, 1991), 146.

10. Menzel, *Strong Medicine*, 29–31.

11. I will not here attempt anything like a justification of AFRP, no mat-

ter which version. It is possible that though AFRP is one of a larger coherent set of principles, there are no more fundamental reasons that can be used to justify it. AFRP might even be needed to explain why any other moral principles bind people: morality as a whole is the collective enterprise, and a reasonable degree of obedience is the fair share everyone is obligated to pay to gain the nonexcludable benefits of morality as a social institution.

12. Menzel, *Strong Medicine,* 30–31.

13. This larger point about the scope of the concept of liberty is made by Amartya Sen, "Liberty and Social Choice," *Journal of Philosophy* 80 (Jan. 1983): 18–20.

14. Failing to recognize that this condition is necessary for presumed prior consent to have any moral force has led several critics to propose very misleading counterexamples to presumed prior consent. See the widget example in Bruce A. Ackerman, "Talking and Trading," *Columbia Law Review* 85 (June 1985): 903, which I discuss in *Strong Medicine,* 31, and the corn subsidy and lottery ticket examples in Daniel Brudney, "Hypothetical Consent and Moral Force," *Law and Philosophy* 10:3 (Aug. 1991): 238–39. In Brudney's lottery ticket example, one comes across an unbelievably good deal on a lottery financed by a philanthropist: 95 percent of the $100 tickets will be redeemed for $10,000. One calls a perfect stranger in the phonebook about investing in a ticket in their name; when one gets no answer, one buys a ticket for the person anyhow. In the immediately subsequent drawing, this ticket turns out to be one of the unlucky 5 percent that lose. Clearly the stranger would have consented to reimburse one $100 for buying them a ticket, yet now one certainly cannot demand that the person pay the $100 when one later tracks them down and explains what one did. A consent that is retrospectively predictable with virtual certainty is morally impotent.

The flaw in using this as a counterexample to presumed prior consent having moral weight, though, ought to be obvious: when we are formulating a workable and efficient policy for who gets lottery tickets, there is no persuasive reason whatsoever for using a prior temporal vantage point for decision making. Watching potential lottery windfalls go unexploited by individuals who are not available when plenty of other eager purchasers are causes us little if any consternation, especially when the activity is an optional one (gambling). Health care coverage is very different. We face an ominous and rapid escalation of costs that virtually everyone in a community (except perhaps providers) has an interest in bringing under control, and getting control at any after-the-fact vantage point is immensely difficult *compared to* gaining consent to restrictions at an earlier point in time.

15. See the book example in Nozick, *Anarchy, State, and Utopia,* 93–94, and the wine bottle example discussed in Menzel, *Strong Medicine,* 30.

16. For explanation, note Menzel, *Strong Medicine,* 32–33.

17. A case before the Fourth Judicial District Court, Hennepin County, Minnesota, from February to July 1991. In addition to miscellaneous newspaper articles during these months, my information on the case is taken from an unpublished but widely distributed detailed communication on the case from S. Miles, M.D., Hennepin County Medical Center, Mar. 22, 1991; Ronald Cranford, "Helga Wanglie's Ventilator," *Hastings Center Report* 21:4 (1991): 23–24; Michael Rie, "The Limits of a Wish," *Hastings Center Report* 21:4 (1991): 24–26; and Felicia Ackerman, "The Significance of a Wish," *Hastings Center Report* 21:4 (1991): 27–29.

18. Ackerman, "Significance of a Wish," 29.

19. The logic here would be that dying patients have an interest in being remembered well by their closest family and friends. See the dissenting opinion by Justice Stevens in *Cruzan v. Missouri Department of Health,* 110 S. Ct. 2841 (1990): 2882.

20. The same strategy can be defended for public insurance coverage, too, I would think. It may be objected that poorer members of a public plan will not have a realistic option of buying up to permanent coma life support coverage, and indeed most do not. Still, how should we think through conceptually where to draw the line of "essential," "basic," or "minimally decent" care that we think a public program is morally obligated to cover? I would argue that it is either by giving the plan's clientele an explicit, direct, or representative vote on the issue, or by hazarding as accurate a judgment as we can about the choice the clientele would make about such coverage if, as informed, rational, and prudent choosers, they could shift resources out of a high-side health care package to meet their other needs. See Menzel, *Strong Medicine,* 126–28.

21. Menzel, "Counting the Costs of Lifesaving Interventions."

22. For an interesting, somewhat modified example of this that has recently provoked controversy, see the case of several utility companies in New Jersey, New York, and New England described by M. Freudenheim, "Utilities Want to Raise Rates to Meet Future Health Costs," *New York Times,* Jan. 7, 1992, A-1, C-20.

23. Nancy S. Jecker, "Age-Based Rationing and Women," *Journal of the American Medical Association* 266 (Dec. 4, 1991): 3012–15.

2

Justice between the Young and the Old
Rationing from an International Perspective

Norman Daniels

Fads, Fashions, and Provincialism

Beginning in the early 1990s, the focus of health policy discussion shifted from concerns about cost-containment, rationing, and the conflicting needs of the young and the old to national health insurance reform aimed at closing the "insurance gap." Ironically, throughout the 1980s, the public was assured that improved access would not be possible without a solution to the problem of rapidly rising health care costs. Nevertheless, although we have failed in all efforts to slow the rate of health cost increases, the public is bombarded with insurance reform proposals, many of which pay little attention, if any, to the burning issues of the 1980s. Were these concerns of the last dozen years, especially as they bear on health policy for the elderly, merely fads and fashions?

The 1980s discussion had three important foci. First, there was concern about the inadequacy of our long-term care system and the need for insurance coverage for this care. Some effort was made to promote "private" solutions, either through appeals to families to "take responsibility" for their elderly (which they already do) or through largely unsuccessful efforts to develop a private insurance market for long-term care (which we have good reason to believe cannot work). Furthermore, public insurance for long-term care (through Medicaid) experienced rapid cost escalation, putting severe pressures on state budgets. The long-term care problem remains unsolved, though some political figures consider it an essential feature of overall health care reform.

The second focus for discussion, on "intergenerational equity," emerged in the mid-1980s. Two complaints were conflated: (1) we under serve the health needs of children, giving too much to the elderly, a problem of distribution between age groups; (2) the current elderly fare much better than the current working population will when it ages, a problem of equity between birth cohorts. Both complaints about intergenerational equity were fueled by demographics and politics. The rapidly growing elderly population seemed a "bottomless pit" of needs, yet the meeting of those needs and financially stabilizing the transfer schemes that fund social security and Medicare required higher taxes at a time when tax increases were political anathema. Some conservatives argued that only privatization of these cash-flow transfer schemes would secure intergenerational equity (every generation supported by its own IRA's).

The third focus of discussion was on rationing health care to the elderly. Since cost containment would in general require explicit rationing, and since the elderly use services at a higher rate than the young, some argued that rationing to the elderly would be a necessary feature of any successful reform. Not surprisingly, this proved the touchiest issue in the health policy arena: Daniel Callahan was vilified for his rationing proposals. The Oregon rationing plan initially dodged the issue by restricting its ranking of services to the non-elderly, non-disabled portion of the Medicaid population, though this strengthened charges by the Children's Defense Fund that the plan was ageist. (There are now plans to extend the ranking to cover the remainder of Medicaid services.)

Although the current national proposals for health care insurance reform have pushed the discussion of health policy for the elderly into the background, we should not be diverted from the issues raised in the 1980s. These issues were rooted in very basic facts about demography and health care needs. If, as I hope, our society comprehensively reforms health care insurance, it will have to embody solutions to these problems. They will not go away until they are dealt with squarely in policy, for the problems raised by the aging of society are not themselves mere fad or fashion. Evidence for this claim can be gleaned by examining, even briefly, what the aging of populations means for health policy elsewhere, both in developed and developing countries. After a brief look at that evidence, I develop an approach to the problems of justice between age groups and birth cohorts and the design of health care institutions.

Population Aging and Health Policy Abroad

Those over age seventy-five or eighty-five are the fastest growing age groups in our population. This is not merely a domestic trend. The elderly population in some northern European countries already constitutes a larger percentage of their population (over 15 percent in some cases) than ours (only about 11 percent). We will not achieve that level of population aging for more than a decade. Moreover, there are parts of Europe where the birth rates have fallen significantly below United States levels. They too must support an aging population when the proportion of the population that works is shrinking. Their health care expenditures must also respond to an aging population and the rapid growth of medical technology. Consequently, European universal access systems are also discussing more openly the need for explicit rationing of health care services. (The Netherlands has had several conferences and a commission devoted to the issue; a WHO conference held in Italy in November 1991 was also partly devoted to the issue of rationing, and a conference in Stockholm on "priorities" is planned for 1996.)

Many developing countries also experience similar issues. Better public health measures have reduced mortality rates, and other social changes have led to lower birth rates. These demographic changes, combined with rapid urbanization and industrialization, mean that the elderly find they can no longer rely on traditional family supports characteristic of agrarian societies. There are fewer children, and many of them move away from their families to work in cities, leaving the elderly behind. Even if they bring their elderly parents with them, the parents can no longer do the kinds of productive work they were able to perform on farms. What is worse, these poor societies must face this crisis without a tradition of any publicly administered transfer scheme from the working population to the elderly. It is ironic, as one Nigerian physician explained to me, that the same appeals to traditional family values that we associated with the Reagan administration are invoked in his country to divert public attention from the need for adequate long-term care policies. (Who wrote the guidebook on how to mislead people?)

This glance abroad supports three claims. First, the underlying forces, demographic, economic, and technological, that drove the U.S. discussion of health care and the elderly in the 1980s are worldwide. Though "closing the insurance gap" is a distinctively American problem, designing a health care system that accommodates changing demographics is not. Second, all countries must openly face the moral issues underlying the explicit rationing of health care. This is true even though some systems have assured universal access and provided better long-term care than we have. Third, we need a very general solution to the problem of justice between age groups and birth cohorts. Any approach that derives solely from features of the U.S. situation, or that focuses on health care in isolation from other manifestations of the problem, or that traces the problem to distinctively American traits ("excessive individualism") is likely to prove inadequate. That is why I turn now to explaining the approach I developed several years ago, defending it against some important objections, and contrasting it with some alternatives.

Welfare Rights and Two Problems of Distributive Justice

Two challenging problems of distributive justice underlie the call for intergenerational equity. First, what is a just or fair distribution of social resources among age groups? According to the Prudential Lifespan Account I sketch, we should count as fair a distribution that prudently allocates a lifetime fair share of a particular resource, such as income support or health care, to each stage of our lives. Second, what is fair treatment of different cohorts as they age and pass through transfer and savings schemes? I believe that our transfer schemes must aim at rough equality in benefit ratios between cohorts. A just arrangement must solve both problems simultaneously. (Because of space limitations, however, I shall say little in what follows about the birth cohort problem.)[1] Of course, solutions to these problems are not all that is involved in producing just social institutions: other intergroup problems of distributive justice must be solved first.

The age group and birth cohort problems have been little discussed in the philosophical literature. Although every society has some system of transfer of wealth, power, and other goods between age groups and birth cohorts, we do not notice these "solutions" to the problems because stable, traditional institutions camouflage them. Rapidly changing economic, social, and demographic conditions expose the problem by forcing new choices about how to satisfy welfare rights.

Articles 23 through 26 of the United Nations Universal Declaration of Human Rights,[2] for example, affirm that people have welfare rights to decent jobs, to rest and leisure, to a standard of living adequate to assure health and well-being, and to education. In a general and abstract way these articles assert that nations have obligations to insure that certain basic human interests and needs are met. What these rights require governments to do or entitle individuals to claim is difficult to enumerate. Often it depends on the needs that must be met and on their distribution in the society. In a rural, agricultural society, the needs of the small number of elderly may be met through part-time employment and family support. The rights of these elderly to a decent standard of living may thus be met through traditional employment patterns and the discharge of familial obligations, without any governmental intervention. (Of course, traditional agricultural societies varied considerably in the degree to which, and the arrangements by which, they met the needs of the elderly; I am not advocating the myth of the pre-modern Golden Age of the family.)[3] But industrialization and urbanization, combined with a major demographic shift that produces large numbers of elderly, may mean that their basic economic needs are no longer met. New social transfer mechanisms must be created or the welfare rights of the elderly will be violated.

Similarly, what a government is obliged to do to meet the health care rights of its citizens depends on the profile of medical needs in that society and on the resources that can be made available to meet those needs. In the same way, what individuals are entitled to claim by way of medical services depends on what counts as a fair distribution of medical services, given those needs and the limitations on resources available to meet them. For example, when there are very few aged people with partial disabilities, and when there are typically many children per aged parent, including adult daughters not in the work force, and when medical technology can rarely prolong the lives of the frail elderly, then their "right to long-term health care" (which seems to be implied by Article 25 of the United Nations Declaration) appears to be satisfied by the discharge of family obligations. But as all these conditions change, social resources for long-term care, including personal services at home, become an important way of meeting health care needs and discharging health care rights. (I am not implying that family support no longer is an important way of meeting personal care needs of the frail elderly in industrialized societies. Families provide about 80 percent of such support in the United States.)[4]

The Prudential Lifespan Account

When is a distribution of resources between the young and the old just? The answer turns on the humbling fact that we all age. In contrast, we do not change sex or race. The relevance of these banal observations needs some explanation.

If we treat blacks and whites or men and women differently, then we produce an inequality between persons, and such inequalities raise questions about justice. For example, if we hire and fire on the basis of race or sex rather than talents and skills, then we create inequalities that are objectionable on grounds of justice. If we treat the old and the young differently, however, we may or may not produce an inequality between persons. If we treat them differently just occasionally and arbitrarily, then we will be treating different persons unequally. But if we treat the young one way as a matter of policy and the old another, and we do so over their whole lives, then we treat all persons equally.

My account of justice between age groups builds on this basic point: unequal treatment at different stages of life may be exactly what we want from institutions that operate over a lifetime. Since our needs vary at different stages of our lives, we want institutions to be responsive to these changes. For example, in many industrialized countries we defer income from our working lives to our post-work retirement period through some combination of individual savings and employee or government pension or social security plan. In many such schemes there are no vested savings, but a direct transfer from the working young to the retired old. Viewed at a moment, it appears that "we" young workers are taxed to benefit "them," the old. If the system is stable over the life span, it appears that our needs for income vary through the different stages of life and we have designed a system that treats us appropriately, that is, differently, at different ages.

The same point holds for health care. When we reach age sixty-five in the United States, we consume health care resources at about 3.5 times the rate (in dollars) that we do prior to age sixty-five. But we pay, as young working people, a combined health care insurance premium—through private premiums, through employee contributions, and through social security taxes—that covers not just our actuarially fair costs, but the health care costs of the elderly and of children as well. Age groups are treated differently. The old pay less and get more, the young pay more and get less. If this system continues as we age, others will pay "inflated premiums" that will cover our higher costs when we are elderly. In effect the system allows us to defer the use of resources from stages in our lives when we need them less into ones in which we need them more. In general, budgeting these transfers prudently enables us to take from some parts of our lives in order to make our lives as a whole better.

We have learned two important lessons about the unequal treatment of different age groups. First, treating the young and old differently does not mean that persons are treated unequally over their life span. Second, unequal treatment of the young and old may have effects that benefit everyone. These two points provide the central intuition behind what I call the Prudential Lifespan Account of justice between age groups: prudent allocation among stages of our lives is our guide to what is just between the young and the old.

The lifespan account involves a fundamental shift of perspective. We must not look at the problem as one of justice between distinct groups in competition with each other, for example, between working adults who pay high premiums and the frail elderly who consume so many services. Rather, we must see that each group represents a stage of our lives. We must view the prudent allocation of resources through the stages of life as our guide to justice between groups. From the perspective of stable institutions operating over time, unequal treatment of people by age appears to be budgeting within a life. If we are concerned with net benefits within a life, we can appeal to a standard principle of individual rational choice: it is rational and prudent that persons take from one stage of their life to give to another in order to make life as a whole better. If the transfers made by an income support or health care system are prudent, they improve individual well-being. Different individuals in such schemes are each made better off, even when the transfers involve unequal treatment of the young and the old. This means that neither old nor young have grounds for complaint that the system is unfair.

Just as individuals set reasonable limits on their lifetime insurance premiums, prudent planners acting on behalf of society in general are limited by what counts as a *fair share* of health care. This share is not simply a dollar allotment per person. It consists of entitlements to services that are contingent on our having certain medical needs. The problem is to find the distributive principle that allocates this fair share over the whole life span. Their goal is a distribution that people in each age group would think is fair because they would all agree it makes their lives as a whole better than alternatives. To insure that our planners avoid biasing the design in favor of their own age group, we shall force them to pretend that they do not know how old they are, and we require that they accept a distribution only if they are willing to live with what it does to them at each stage of their lives. Each stage of their own lives thus stands in as proxy for an age group, and they will age from conception to death in the system of trade-offs to which they agree.

It is important to contrast the Prudential Lifespan Account sketched here with Menzel's insurance account of rationing presented in the preceding chapter. My deliberators depart more than Menzel's from the model of the fully rational and informed deliberator. For example, I block information about how old we are. I also block other information that might give too much weight to our current plan of life or preferences.[5] More than that, I restrict the role of prudence to deliberation about how to allocate a *lifetime fair share* of health care, where that share is what results when institutions are governed by a principle protecting equality of opportunity. The appeal to prudence already presupposes that justice prevails in the distribution of goods between groups of people. The appeal to prudence to solve the age group problem is thus "framed" by other considerations of justice. In contrast, Menzel believes that no such frame is necessary and that prudent insurers, thinking ex ante about health care benefits over the life span, can specify what counts as a just distribution of health care. I reject Menzel's more general appeal to prudent insurers because prudence alone cannot tell us which distributions are fair when they cross boundaries between persons. This difference in our view produces significantly different outcomes. For example, if my Prudential Lifespan Account justifies a health care policy or social security policy that has differential impact on people by race, class, or gender, then the policy may have to be reconsidered. It will have violated the requirements of the "frame." But Menzel's account involves no such constraint.

Generality of the Prudential Lifespan Account

Before outlining what the Prudential Lifespan Account specifically implies for health policy, I want to emphasize its applicability to welfare rights more generally. For example, Article 25 of the Human Rights Declaration includes rights to income support during periods of unemployment, including retirement in old age. The young and the old seem to be in competition here just as much as in the case of health care. The Prudential Lifespan Account asks us to think about how planners who do not know their age would allocate a lifetime fair share of such entitlements to each stage of life. Here, too, the lifetime fair share is not some lump sum in dollars but a range of contingent entitlements to support. These entitlements are specified relative to what justice in general permits in the way of economic inequalities between persons.

Prudent planners, operating under the constraints I have sketched before, would have to reason as follows about such entitlements to support. They cannot expand their lifetime income share by allocating it in certain ways, for example by setting aside income early in life and investing it heavily in their own human capital or otherwise. Such investment strategies are already accommodated within the notion of a lifetime fair income share, or so I am supposing when I imagine them budgeting a fixed but fair lifetime share. (At the level of resources it is a zero sum game, though the resource can be allocated in ways that can be estimated to make their lives go better or worse overall.) These planners do not know how old they are, and they must allow for the fact that their preferences or views about what is good in life will change over the life span. The prudent course of action would be to allocate their fair share in such a way that standard of living would remain roughly equal over the life span (call this the Standard of Living Preservation Principle). They would want institutions to facilitate income transfers over the life span in such a way that individuals have available to themselves, at each stage of life, an adequate income to pursue whatever plan they may at that stage . Of course, "adequate" is here relative to the individual's fair income share, as determined by the acceptable inequalities in the society. This principle has implications for income support in old age.

The Prudential Lifespan Account can also be used to help us think about the general rights to education described in Article 26 of the Human Rights Declaration. We are used to thinking of education as a process early in life, one that helps set the trajectory for the quality of later life. But as more and more people live longer lives in the context of rapidly changing technologies, and as societies age, we must think anew about the role of education throughout the life span.

The generality of the Prudential Lifespan Account is, I believe, one of its virtues. Its strengths and weaknesses should be assessed independently of the merits of the account of justice we might offer for the particular goods, like health care, to which it can be applied.[6] It is *general* in two ways: it applies to various goods, not just health care, and it tells us about rationing goods across the life span, not just about age-based rationing. Before turning to my use of the approach in health care and in arguments about rationing health care by age, I want to consider some objections that have been raised to the Prudential Lifespan Account in general.

Some Objections

One objection raised to the Prudential Lifespan Account is that its application can create some intergroup inequalities. This objection must be taken seriously because the rationale for adopting the prudential model for the age group problem is that we can assume that intra-life transfers will be an appropriate model for inter-age-group transfers, but if different demographic groups age differently, then the modeling breaks down. A good example is that raising the age of eligibility for income support benefits under Social Security—which arguably is a prudent and fair way to address both the age group and birth cohort problems—might leave African Americans, who have lower life expectancy, worse off than whites or Asians. Similarly, a policy of rationing by age, which is permissible under certain conditions of scarcity on my account, might have differential impact by class, race, or gender. Where such effects take place, they might constitute reasons for not adopting such a rationing policy, or they might give us reasons to link the rationing to facts about group life expectancy. The general point is that the Prudential Lifespan Account presupposes that solutions to the age group problem will not disturb more general requirements of justice.

One very interesting objection to my account is raised by McKerlie,[7] who questions the adequacy of what he calls the "complete lives" version of egalitarianism it seems to rest on. Treating people differently at different ages, I argued, does not always create an inequality that requires justification if we judge from the perspective of their complete lives. In contrast, treating people differently by race or sex does create such inequalities over complete lives. McKerlie, building on some suggestions of Parfit,[8] claims that the complete lives view has puzzling and unacceptable consequences. Consider two. Suppose A's life has been worse than B's (say A had a poor childhood), but A is not scarred by his past. Complete lives egalitarianism seems to imply we should favor A in the future to compensate for his past deficits, but it is not obvious that our egalitarian intuitions would support making B worse off than A in the future to accomplish this. Similarly, imagine a feudal society that contains nobles and peasants who switch places every ten years. Over their whole lives, they are equally happy, but at each time slice significant inequalities exist. If no basic rights are violated by the arrangement, complete lives egalitarianism seems unable to explain what seems wrong with the significant inequalities switching places produces between simultaneous segments of lives.

Contrary to McKerlie's suggestion, however, I have not intended the appeal to complete lives as a complete account of our egalitarian inclinations. Rather, I invoke the complete lives view for a specific, limited purpose. My goal is to develop an account of how we should think about the design of social institutions that distribute goods over the whole of our lives. I construe the problem of institutional design as an answer to the question, how should we ex ante want such distributive schemes to treat us at each stage of life? Because stable policies that treat people differently at different ages do not generate the same objectionable inequalities that sexist or racist treatment produce over complete lives, they do not face a crucial objection raised by sexist or racist treatment. More to the point, in my view not every inequality between segments of lives is acceptable just because the complete lives are equal. I also require that the differential treatment we permit between stages of life is prudent; inequalities between segments must work to make our lives go as well as possible, given the limits imposed by the lifetime fair share of resources (generally, I am talking about resource inequalities between stages of life, not utility inequalities). Since the switching between nobles and peasants is unlikely to be prudent, it is not acceptable on my account.[9]

Health Care and the Prudential Lifespan Account

Consider now how the Prudential Lifespan Account might be applied to the case of health care. To see what the account means, we must characterize our lifetime fair share of health care in a principled way. To specify this notion, we must show in general what principle of distributive justice should govern the design of the health care system. Our fair share will be the services we have contingent claims on, given that institutions are designed in accordance with that principle.

I have argued elsewhere that a central, unifying function of health care is to maintain and restore functioning that is typical or normal for our species.[10] Health care derives its moral importance from the following fact: normal functioning has a central effect on the opportunity open to an individual. It helps guarantee individuals a fair chance to enjoy the normal opportunity range for their society. The normal opportunity range for a given society is the array of life plans reasonable persons in it are likely to construct for themselves. Individuals' fair share of the normal opportunity range is the array of life plans they may reasonably choose, given their talents and skills. Disease and disability shrinks that share from what is fair; health care protects it. The suggestion that emerges from this account is that we should use impairment of the normal opportunity range as a fairly crude measure of the relative moral importance of health care needs at the macro level.

Because we have obligations to assure people fair equality of opportunity, we have social obligations to provide health care services that protect and restore normal functioning. This account implies that there should be no financial, geographical, or discriminatory barriers to a level of care that promotes normal functioning, given reasonable or necessary limits on resources. We can guide hard public policy choices about which services are more important to provide by considering their relative impact on the normal opportunity range. Rights to health care are thus *system relative:* entitlements to services can only be specified within a system that works to protect opportunity as well as possible, given limited resources.

Our prudent planners solve the age group problem if they can clarify what the right to health care means for each age group. To do this, they must agree to a principle for allocating their lifetime fair share to each stage of life. (A crucial contrast with Menzel's approach is this characterization of the fair share that we must prudently allocate over the life span.) Remember, these planners do not know how old they are. This means that it is especially important for them to make sure social arrangements give them a chance to enjoy their fair share of the normal range of opportunities open to them at each stage of life. This protection of opportunity at each stage of life is particularly important, since they are planning for their whole lives and must keep in mind the importance of being able to revise their views about what is valuable in life as they age. But impairments of normal functioning by disease and disability clearly restrict the portion of the normal opportunity range open to individuals at any stage of their lives. Consequently, health care services should be rationed throughout a life in a way that respects the importance of the age-relative normal opportunity range. In effect, all specific allocation decisions must be constrained by this principle.

Health Policy Implications of the Prudential Lifespan Account

Long-Term Care

Because the likelihood of needing long-term care increases with age, the aging of society raises urgent questions about the long-term care systems in many developed countries. Some experts suggest that long-term care "may well be the major health and social issue of the next four decades, polarizing society over the next twenty to forty years."[11] By 2040 there is likely to be a fivefold increase in the number of people aged eighty-five and over. There will be similar increases in the numbers of very old who are nursing home residents or functionally dependent.[12] These trends are present in both developed and developing countries. In some countries the absence of existing public long-term care systems magnifies the problem.

Long-term care, I have argued, is of comparable moral importance to acute care.[13] They have the same function, protecting an individual's share of the normal opportunity range. Although long-term care services are sometimes defended as cost-saving measures (which they may not always be), and sometimes on the grounds that they preserve dignity, it is their impact on the range of opportunities open to an individual that is more basic. I believe it is this impact that explains the importance of these services to preserving self-respect.[14]

By adding the perspective of the Prudential Lifespan Account, two further points can be made. It may be prudent to trade some acute care services aimed at marginal extension of life for long-term care services that greatly improve quality of life over a longer period. Second, providing public long-term care services can bring relief to families providing this care privately. This provides a benefit at two stages of life—when we are providers of such care and when we receive it. The suggestion that emerges from these considerations is that the U.S. system has undervalued the importance of long-term care and under-supplied crucial services that benefit us at various points in the life span. Any redesign of our health care insurance system should include reallocation of benefits reflecting these priorities.

In some universal access systems, like the Canadian and some European systems, long-term care services, including many social support and home services, are already incorporated in the benefit package. Rationing health care in these systems will require making explicit the way in which the importance of these services are measured against the importance of existing and forthcoming acute care technologies. We have not developed an adequate philosophical framework for thinking about how to make these judgments in any very specific manner. I take this to be a crucial problem for the 1990s that bears on health care rationing and the elderly. The Oregon Health Services Commission faces this problem as it attempts to expand the ranking of services to include services for the elderly and disabled.

One useful lesson for developing countries is to avoid the bias that exists in many developed countries in favor of high technology acute care and against long-term care services. A number of commentators have emphasized the importance of facilitating the care of the elderly by paying attention to housing and other community policies that allow families to preserve support relationships in nontraditional settings.[15] These are promising alternatives, but they require positive steps to be taken by government, and they are not to be confused with simply allowing traditional family supports to continue, for the economic and social fabric surrounding that support has been altered.

Rationing by Age

In the United States there is considerable concern that the increasing numbers of elderly will intensify the problem of rapidly rising health care costs. Much of this rate of increase is due to the rapid dissemination of high cost medical technologies, many of which are aimed at conditions that are prevalent among the elderly. In this context there is a growing discussion about the need to ration beneficial medical treatments. In the United States the greatest threat to health care rights will come from the temptation to use ability to pay as a criterion for rationing, but there is a growing discussion of the relevance of age as a basis for rationing some high cost medical technologies. Callahan has drawn considerable critical comment for his proposal that we consider rationing life extending medical services explicitly by age.[16] Less hypothetically, there is evidence that the British National Health Service already uses age as a basis for rationing some expensive technologies, such as renal dialysis,[17] and in the United

States many transplants are not made available to people over age fifty-five. The explanation usually given, that they will not do as well as younger people, appears to have little in the way of controlled studies to support it.

Some critics of rationing by age consider it morally impermissible in exactly the way that rationing by race or sex would be. They consider age, as opposed to medical suitability, a "morally irrelevant" basis for distributing medical services. Others advocate a policy of rationing by age because they believe that the elderly have a duty to step aside and sacrifice for the young.[18] Still others believe that it is fair for the elderly, who have had the opportunity to live a long time, to forego services in favor of the young, who have had less opportunity to live.[19]

The Prudential Lifespan Account provides a way to resolve this dispute.[20] Would prudent planners ever have a reason to prefer (or not to reject) rationing by age? Under some conditions of resource scarcity they would. Suppose that making a scarce life-extending resource available to everyone who needs it regardless of age means that it is less available to the young. Then the young will have a reduced chance of reaching normal life expectancy, while the old will have an increased chance of living to a ripe old age. Prudent planners who do not know how old they are might then have reason to ration such technologies by age, making them more available to the young than to the very old. More precisely, if we consider only information about life-years saved, and if rationing by age and rationing by lottery both yield the same life expectancy, it is not imprudent to prefer an increased chance of reaching that life expectancy through age rationing. If we add more information, for example, that years later in life are more likely to contain disabilities, or that years earlier in life are typically more important to carrying out central projects in life, then we can get the stronger result that age rationing is preferred to rationing by lottery. Judging from the perspective of a whole life, not only is each person treated equally despite the age rationing, but each person is better off.

This argument turns on no prior moral assumptions that life at one age is more *valuable* than life at another. It does not turn on the judgment that it is more important or valuable for society to save the young than the old or that society would benefit more from doing so. Instead it turns on the judgment each of us would in effect make, that we would each be better off (or no worse off) from an age rationing scheme. Nor does it turn on prior moral views about the duties of the elderly to the young or vice versa.

It is a virtue of this argument that it does not invoke prior moral judgments of any of these kinds. Contrast it, for example, with Brock's suggestion (similar to Veatch's)[21] that we should simply and directly invoke the principle of equality of opportunity. It tells us, he claims, that we better assure equality of opportunity if we give everyone a better chance of reaching normal life expectancy (through age rationing) than if we allow unequal chances of reaching normal life expectancy (through a straight lottery). I am not claiming that Brock (or Veatch) is wrong about what our intuitions about equality of opportunity imply. I am, however, reluctant to appeal to them in so straightforward a way. Does it matter, for example, whether an old person in need of such services had never been a beneficiary of earlier medical assistance, or whether a younger person had many resources devoted to their protection? Just what factors do our intuitions here turn on? Part of what is at issue is whether we should judge the equality of opportunity as assured by the outcome (more equal chances at achieving normal life expectancy) or by a process (more equal chances through a lottery at receiving the life-extending service). I think that our intuitions pull in different directions on this matter. My prudential argument, however, makes no such appeal to such intuitions.

The contrast with Callahan's argument for rationing by age is also striking, for his turns crucially on claims about moral obligations that play no role in mine. I believe the overall structure of Callahan's argument can be captured in the following three-step argument:

1. The only way life for the old is meaningful is if the old serve the young.
2. The old ought to serve the young, for example, by serving as moral exemplars who surrender claims on lifesaving services in favor of the young.
3. The old can be compelled through age-rationing measures to carry out their obligations to the young.

This argument is both unsound and invalid. There is no one way for the old to find meaning in their lives. Of course, serving the young might be one way. But there are other ways for the old to find meaning in their lives. (Claude Pepper, for example, found meaning in his old age by serving the old.) In a culturally diverse society we are likely to differ considerably in our views about what adds meaning to old age. Similarly, if we look at other cultures—which, as I noted earlier, face the same problems of population aging—we are likely to find quite varied views about the meaning of life in old age. Indeed, some cultures might reach exactly the opposite conclusion to the one reached by Callahan. If Callahan's appeal to "communitarianism" is to be taken seriously, then his hope that we can instill his view about meaningful old age in our culture, or make it dominant in other societies, is unlikely. Under this commitment to communitarianism, it is hard to see how he can reject community affirmation of values that oppose his view of the duty of the elderly.

Suppose, for the sake of argument, that Callahan's first premise (above) is true. Then the argument fails because we cannot derive the second step from it, nor the third step from the second step. From the fact that something makes my life meaningful, it does not follow that it is what I *ought* to do or seek. Many things might add meaning to my life, but they are things I am not obliged to do on either prudential or moral grounds. Moreover, many of the things I ought to do are not things that society should compel me to do, which is the force of the conclusion of the argument.

Whereas Callahan puts his argument to use as a rationale for a general policy, I do not advocate age rationing as a policy. My argument supports age rationing only under very particular conditions in which scarcity has a distinctive effect. My argument also defends age rationing only by showing that it may be more prudent than a straight lottery. If (as I believe) there are alternative strategies for allocating resources, for example, ones more fine-tuned to the conditions of patients and the likely outcomes of treating them, then rationing by age may prove less prudent than these alternatives, and the Prudential Lifespan Account would not approve of age rationing. In contrast, there is considerable unclarity regarding just what role scarcity or cost-containment plays in Callahan's argument. He prefaces his discussion with concerns about rising health care costs and claims about scarcity, but the argument itself (as sketched above) does not appeal to scarcity. Nor does Callahan show just what the savings would be if his policy was adopted (Schwartz and Aaron argue there would be very minor savings at best).[22]

I have already alluded to the fact that solutions to the age group problem must fit within solutions to more general problems of distributive justice, for example, between groups that cannot be thought of as sharing a life span. The point holds for rationing by age: its acceptability must be weighed against any intergroup inequalities it creates, for example, between classes, races, or genders. Other constraints of justice also apply. Rationing, I have elsewhere argued, must be public both with regard to the criteria used and the rationale for employing them and must be agreed upon through democratic processes.[23] My suspicion is that the use of age-based rationing in the British National Health Service would not survive public scrutiny, in part because the rationale that has emerged for it ("the elderly patients are too crumbly") would not survive.

Given all these constraints, it seems quite likely that other criteria for rationing medical services would seem preferable to pure age-based rationing, especially since such rationing is justifiable, in my view, only under very special circumstances. To show that age-based rationing meets the requirement that resources be scarce in the way demanded by my argument, we would have to show (except for some naturally scarce resources) that other alternatives, including more stringent general rationing, would not eliminate the effects of the scarcity. That is a condition it would be very difficult to meet when more general forms of rationing have not been tried.

Before developed countries with comprehensive, universal health care systems can undertake explicit, publicly defensible rationing, they must address three central moral issues: (1) When shall we depart from giving people equal chances at some important benefit (survival, reduced disability) because someone else has a better outcome or chance of success? (2) When shall we give priority to meeting the needs of someone with a less serious condition rather than someone with a more serious condition? (3) When shall we give priority to meeting the lesser needs of greater numbers of people rather than the more serious needs of smaller numbers of people? My recommendation is that philosophers dedicate themselves to these more general problems rather than attempting to show just when rationing by age would be a clearly defensible policy.

I might add that in developing countries the issue of age-based rationing should be even further from the public agenda. The reason is that the real rationing problems in these countries involve resisting efforts to displace health care budgets aimed at providing adequate preventive and primary care in favor of acute care services that are likely to be used only by the wealthiest sectors of the population. From an international perspective, despite the prominence of the aging of populations as a social issue, rationing health care by age remains a largely diversionary proposal. In general, it is very likely that there are better strategies for rationing health care than rationing by age—ones that would be judged preferable by the Prudential Lifespan Account.

A More General Problem about Rationing

In applying the Prudential Lifespan Account to health care, I claim that we should protect equality of opportunity at each stage of life. But since resources are limited we must make choices that sometimes mean we will protect the normal opportunity range better at one stage of life than another. Yet nothing in my theory tells us specifically how to make such choices. My account is seriously incomplete.[24] But the problem is really quite general and amounts to a criticism about most nonutilitarian accounts of distributive justice. At the risk of digression, let me develop the general point, at least programmatically.[25]

We tend to think of rationing as an exceptional practice responding to unusual scarcity, for example, the wartime use of coupons for gasoline, waiting lists for bodily organs, or battlefield triage. Philosophers have generally thought these practices peripheral to the central problems of distributive justice. In fact, however, rationing is a common, quite central practice. We ration whenever we design institutions and policies that embody our concerns about distributive justice under ordinary resource limitations. Viewed in this light, many examples of rationing come to mind: raising eligibility standards for welfare, job training programs, or Medicaid; funding public defenders or "reasonable accommodations" for the disabled; determining the ratio of learning disability specialists to "mainstream" teachers. We must often deny benefits to some who can plausibly claim they are owed them in principle. A general account of the ethical issues involved in rationing, broadly construed, would provide a "missing link" in ethical theory.

Our beliefs about justice commonly tell us we must distribute important goods in accord with specific principles. For instance, we might think that health care or legal defense should be distributed according to need and not ability to pay. Nevertheless, resources are inadequate to meet all the claims individuals legitimately seem to have on these goods. We simply cannot afford to educate, treat medically, or protect legally in all the ways people can plausibly claim to need. There is another level of decision making—it concerns who gets what when all can cite the principles on their behalf. Moreover, unlike money, the goods that we can provide in each domain are not sufficiently divisible to avoid unequal or "lumpy" distributions. For example, we cannot divide an organ: if one gets it, another does not. Or, if we introduce legal aid for criminal but not civil legal defense, some groups fare better than others.

Principles of distributive justice alone are thus not adequate to establish which policies or institutions are just. Rawls suggests that the problem is ultimately a legislative one.[26] Adequately informed legislators, sensitive to conflicting claims, will design institutions that embody principles of distributive justice. Are these legislative decisions constrained by principles of rationing, however? A theory of rationing would constitute a crucial *bridge* between different levels of reasoning about justice. We need such an account whether we believe, like Rawls and Gauthier, in a general theory of distributive justice, or, like Walzer, only in principles of distributive justice that are specific to "spheres."[27]

A theory of rationing would have to answer several general questions. First, when is it appropriate to rely on a *fair process,* such as a lottery or a publicly accountable democratic agency, to determine a fair rationing outcome, and when does fair rationing require some *pattern of outcomes,* perhaps reflecting the irreducible content of a particular distributive principle? For example, can we rely on a democratic commission to establish relevant priorities among health care needs, as in the Oregon rationing plan, or is that commission constrained to choose among certain patterns of outcome, for example, giving priority to more serious conditions? Second, when is it reasonable or fair to depart from giving equally needy people *equal chances* at a scarce good (e.g., an organ) in order to promote *better outcomes* from the use of that good? Broome suggests that the plausibility of appealing to random selection in such cases varies with the kind of good being distributed, but he offers no more general characterization of the cases in which it is more and less plausible.[28] Third, how much priority must we give to those whose need is greater when we ration benefits? When should we forego giving a modest benefit to someone whose need is great in order to give a greater benefit to someone whose need is less? Fourth, when may we *aggregate the benefits* from a rationing scheme so that meeting a major educational or medical need of relatively few people may be outweighed by providing for the less important needs of a larger number of people? This question is sometimes cast as if it turned on a choice between utilitarian and more specific distributive principles, but the lumpiness of distribution raises the issue even within a domain governed by a nonutilitarian distributive principle. The theory of rationing is thus a prolegomenon to useful work in crucial areas of applied ethics, including health care rationing.

Conclusion

I have tried to offer a unifying—if abstract—vision of how to solve the problem of intergenerational equity. We all pass through institutions that distribute goods over our life span. If these institutions are prudently designed, we each benefit throughout our lives. It is only prudent to treat ourselves differently at different stages of life, as our needs change. What is prudent with respect to different stages of a life determines what is fair between age groups. Prudence here guides justice. If as policy makers, planners, and the general public we all keep our eye on this unifying vision, and if we can ignore the divisive talk about competition between age groups and birth cohorts, then our target will be policies that benefit us all over our whole lives. Establishing such policies would mean doing justice to the old and the young. It would mean giving clear content to our welfare rights.

Notes

This essay is based in part on material contained in my book *Am I My Parents' Keeper? An Essay on Justice between the Young and the Old* (New York: Oxford University Press, 1988); I thank the publishers for permission to draw on that material here. Some points made here are also to be found in my essay "Human Rights, Population Aging, and Intergenerational Equity," in *Population and Human Rights: Proceedings of the Expert Group Meeting on Population and Human Rights, Geneva, 3–6 April 1989* (New York: United Nations, 1990), 207–30.

1. See Norman Daniels, *Am I My Parents' Keeper?: An Essay on Justice between the Young and the Old* (New York: Oxford University Press, 1988); see also Daniels, "Human Rights, Population Aging, and Intergenerational Equity," in *Population and Human Rights: Proceedings of the Expert Group Meeting on Population and Human Rights, Geneva, 3–6 April 1989* (New York: United Nations, 1990), 207–30.

2. United Nations Universal Declaration of Human Rights, 1948.

3. Daniels, *Am I My Parents' Keeper?* chap. 2; P. Laslett, ed., *Household and Family in Past Time* (Cambridge: Cambridge University Press, 1972); P. Laslett, "Societal Development and Aging," in R. H. Binstock and E. Shanas, eds., *Handbook of Aging and the Social Sciences* (New York: Van Nostrand Reinhold, 1976), 87–160.

4. D. L. Frankfather, M. J. Smith, and F. G. Caro, *Family Care of the Elderly* (Lexington, Mass.: Lexington Books, 1981).

5. See Daniels, *Am I My Parents' Keeper?* chap. 3.

6. See Norman Daniels, "The Biomedical Model and Just Health Care," *Journal of Medicine and Philosophy* 14:6 (1989): 677–80, in response to a criticism by Nancy Jecker in "Towards a Theory of Age-Group Justice," *Journal of Medicine and Philosophy* 14:6 (1989): 655–76.

7. Dennis McKerlie, "Equality between Age Groups," *Philosophy and Public Affairs* 32:3 (1992): 275–95.

8. D. Parfit, *Reasons and Persons* (Oxford: Oxford University Press, 1984), 149–58; D. Parfit, "Comments," *Ethics* 96 (1986): 869–70.

9. See Norman Daniels, "The Prudential Lifespan Account of Justice across Generations," in Lee Cohen, ed., *Justice across Generations: What Does It Mean?* (Washington, D.C.: AARP, 1993), 197–214; and Daniels, "The Prudential Lifespan Account: Objections and Replies," in Cohen, ed., *Justice across Generations*, 243–47.

10. Norman Daniels, *Just Health Care* (Cambridge: Cambridge University Press, 1985).

11. R. J. Vogel and H. C. Palmer, eds., *Long-Term-Care: Perspectives from Research and Demonstrations* (Washington, D.C.: Health Care Financing Administration, U.S. Dept. of Health and Human Services, 1982), v.

12. G. J. Soldo and K. G. Manton, "Changes in the Health Status and Service Needs of the Oldest Old: Current Patterns and Future Trends," *Milbank Memorial Fund Quarterly: Health and Society* 63:2 (1985): 286.

13. Daniels, *Am I My Parents' Keeper?*

14. See Nancy Jecker, "Care for the Disabled Elderly: The Economics of Financing Long-Term Care (chap. 4 in this volume), for an elaboration of this point.

15. M. Powell Lawton, "Environments and Living Arrangements," in R. H. Binstock, W.-S. Chow, and J. H. Schultz, eds., *International Perspectives on Aging: Population and Policy Challenges* (New York: United Nations Fund for Population Activities, 1982), 159–92.

16. Daniel Callahan, *Setting Limits: Medical Goals in an Aging Society* (New York: Simon and Schuster, 1987).

17. H. Aaron and W. Schwartz, *The Painful Prescription* (Washington, D.C.: Brookings Institution, 1984).

18. Lawton, "Environments and Living Arrangements."

19. Robert Veatch, "Justice and the Economics of Terminal Illness," *Hastings Center Report* 18:4 (1988): 34–40; D. Brock, "Ethical Issues in Recipient Selection for Organ Transplantation," in D. Mathieu, ed., *Organ Substitution Technology: Ethical, Legal, and Public Policy Issues* (Boulder: Westview Press, 1988), 86–99.

20. See also Daniels, *Just Health Care,* chap. 5, and *Am I My Parents' Keeper?* chap. 5.

21. Brock, "Ethical Issues in Recipient Selection"; Veatch, "Justice and the Economics of Terminal Illness."

22. William Schwartz and Henry Aaron, "A Tough Choice on Health Care Costs," *New York Times,* Apr. 6, 1988, A23.

23. Norman Daniels, "Is the Oregon Rationing Plan Fair?" *Journal of the American Medical Association* 265:17 (1991): 2232–35; and Daniels, "Rationing Fairly: Programmatic Considerations," *Bioethics* 7:2–3 (1993): 224–33.

24. E. J. Emanuel notes this problem in *The Ends of Human Life: Medical Ethics in a Liberal Polity* (Cambridge: Harvard University Press, 1991), 129ff.

25. See Daniels, "Rationing Fairly."

26. John Rawls, *A Theory of Justice* (Cambridge: Harvard University Press, 1971).

27. D. Gauthier, *Morals by Agreement* (Oxford: Clarendon Press, 1986); M. Walzer, *Spheres of Justice* (New York: Basic Books, 1983).

28. J. Broome, "Selecting People Randomly," *Ethics* 95 (Oct. 1984): 38–55.

Part 2

Applications

3

Is There a Place for Euthanasia in America's Care for Its Elderly?

Margaret P. Battin

Is there a place for euthanasia in America's care for its elderly? Why does this question arise,[1] and why does it seem so provocative? Why might we be asking this question at this particular moment in time? Why can't the answer be just a simple *yes* or *no?*

Presuppositions of the Question

The question of euthanasia and the elderly arises within a specific sociotemporal context—increasing concern over humanitarian issues in medicine, against the background of the cost crisis in health care—but the very posing of the question at all brings with it a number of presuppositions. These presuppositions, often overlooked as we approach the question, include the following five. We can hardly be clear about the answer to the question until we are alert to the assumptions it brings along with it.

A first, and central, presupposition is that the issue of euthanasia and the elderly is a *national* issue—that it is meaningful to speak of "America's" care for its elderly, rather than merely the care provided, say, by specific health providers, institutions, insurers, family members, and so on. Thus it raises questions of policy at the highest level. The question is no longer the local question of whether, for example, you may request euthanasia for yourself when you contract a painful terminal illness or reach old age, or whether you may perform euthanasia for your aged grandmother or ask her physician to do so, or whether her physician may perform euthanasia for her, or even whether a given health care institution or type of institution, such as nursing homes, may ever practice euthanasia. The question, as it reflects the concerns of this country at this point in time, is whether euthanasia should be permitted *as national policy* or, indeed, established as a part of national policy.

At the moment there is only one country in the world in which permitting euthanasia (and physician-assisted suicide) has, in effect, attained the status of national policy: the Netherlands. Dutch policy recognizes voluntary choices of euthanasia and physician-assisted suicide in a range of circumstances. Although these practices remain technically illegal, the physician performing them is protected from prosecution if they meet an established set of guidelines, including not only the requirement that the request be voluntary on the part of the patient and that the patient's choice be considered and stable, but that the patient have adequate information, that the patient be facing intolerable suffering, that the physician have tried all alternatives for relieving the suffering that are acceptable to the patient, and that the physician have consulted with another physician of independent judgment.[2] Whether U.S. policy concerning euthanasia or physician-assisted suicide (though at the moment most discussion in the United States distinguishes fairly sharply between the two, and supports only the latter) would resemble the Dutch policy remains an open issue;[3] what is important here is to see that the assigned question appears to presuppose that, as in the Netherlands, it is national— not merely personal, local, or regional—policy with which we would be concerned. National policy would, of course, require support not only from the law and the courts, but from the medical profession and many other parties as well.

The second presupposition of the question concerning euthanasia and the elderly is that if the question concerning euthanasia were to be answered affirmatively, euthanasia would be one among other components of America's care for its elderly. There would be "*a* place for euthanasia," but euthanasia would not be the only policy in effect. The way the question is posed thus raises the issue of what these alternatives might be: would it be euthanasia vs. full health care? euthanasia vs. limited treatment? euthanasia vs. rationing-based disqualification for treatment, or what? We can hardly consider whether there should be "*a*" place for euthanasia in our treatment of the elderly unless we know what alternatives might be available to the elderly instead; thus this is not a question that can be answered in a theoretical vacuum.

The third presupposition in asking whether there is a place for euthanasia in America's care for the elderly is that care is to be provided by some party other than the elderly, and, hence, that the elderly are not to be expected to—or left to—care for themselves. This is a crucial assumption, but one not always true. For example, the Catastrophic Health Insurance Act of 1990, hastily enacted and even more hastily repealed, involved a funding mechanism that would have expanded health care coverage among the elderly but required financing for the program from the elderly themselves: as "gray power" groups pointed out in opposing the program, it was not a matter of "providing" care for the elderly, but of forcing the elderly to assume the burden of care for themselves. As the issue is raised in the question considered here, it is not a matter of permitting or expecting the elderly to provide euthanasia for themselves; that is, it is not just a question about amateur or self-help euthanasia by the elderly for themselves. Rather, it is a matter of "America"—that is, all age groups in the United States—permitting or providing euthanasia for persons for the most part older than themselves.

The fourth presupposition is that euthanasia can be viewed as an "elderly" issue. However, euthanasia proposals in the United States, including Washington state's Initiative 119 and California's Proposition 161, respectively defeated at the polls in 1991 and 1992 (both by 46 to 54 percent margins), and Oregon's Measure 16 (permitting only physician-assisted suicide), which won by a 51 to 49 percent margin at the polls in November 1994 but has been under continuous legal challenge since then, as well as legislative proposals and public initiatives introduced or in the planning stages in a variety of other states, are exclusively framed as legislation about the terminally ill, not the elderly. The various items of legislation proposed to legalize voluntary active euthanasia and physician-assisted suicide[4] would all apply only to people diagnosed as terminally ill, defined as being within six months of death. The elderly would be ineligible unless also terminally ill. Furthermore, given the information available about euthanasia where it is openly practiced—the Netherlands—it does not seem to be primarily a practice of the elderly. On the contrary, according to the first full-scale empirical studies of euthanasia in the Netherlands, of the approximately 2,300 cases of euthanasia occurring in general practice per year, the average age of the patients involved was sixty-two for men, sixty-six for women; 38 percent of patients receiving euthanasia were younger than sixty-five; only 25 percent were eighty or older.[5] Thus the question of euthanasia for the elderly harbors a radical extension of the discussion, previously confined to terminal illness, not old age.

The fifth presupposition of the question, the last to be considered here, is that the issue is confined to *active* euthanasia. There are two reasons why this presupposition is embedded in the question. First, in ordinary, public discourse, the term "euthanasia" is virtually always used to refer to active euthanasia—direct termination of the patient's life, that is, direct killing—while by and large only philosophers use the expression "passive" euthanasia to refer to withholding and withdrawing treatment. This linguistic fact underlies the second reason: it is assumed that active euthanasia can be discussed intelligibly without reference to passive euthanasia, that is, that the two are distinct phenomena and can be addressed independently. Thus, it is supposed, in asking about euthanasia for the elderly, we can ask this question just about whether the elderly may receive direct, deliberate life-terminating treatment, without also inquiring—as we shall later do—about indirect, semi-intentional ways they may be allowed to die.

Equivocation and the Language of the Question

Even when the principal presuppositions of the question, "Is there a place for euthanasia in America's care for its elderly?" have been teased out—that it is about national policy, that euthanasia would be one among other components of care, that euthanasia would be provided for the elderly by others and they would not have to do it themselves, that euthanasia would not be confined to the terminally ill, and that it is active euthanasia that is at issue—it is still not clear exactly what question is being asked. For the very term "euthanasia" is understood in widely differing ways, and the question cannot be clear until we know which one is at issue. It is crucial to disentangle these two senses—for the most part inconsistently and chaotically used in current disputes about euthanasia—to see how the question looks in this clearer light.

Two distinct senses of active euthanasia seem to be current. On the one hand, there is the sense, based heavily on the Greek root *eu-thanatos,* or "good death," that euthanasia is in the interests of the person whose death it is; it is humane death—a good death, or at least better than the death this person would otherwise meet. In the Netherlands, "euthanasia" is widely understood in this way, and there is an additional component: it is also understood that the wish of the patient is central, and that an actively caused death that is not in concert with the wish of the patient cannot be a good one. Hence, in the Netherlands, "euthanasia" is understood *by definition* to presuppose that it is voluntary euthanasia, or as the authors of the Remmelink Commission report put it, "the intentional termination of life by somebody other than the person concerned at his or her request."[6] The request of the patient "is at the core of the definition of euthanasia."[7] This is not to say that other cases of medical termination do not go on in the Netherlands; they do, but they are generally not described as "euthanasia"; the alternative term usually employed for them is *levensbeeindigend handelen,* or "life-ending treatment without explicit request" (LAWER). Even these cases are practiced just where there has been an informal advance request ("Doctor, if it ever gets too bad, please do something") or where the patient is suffering severely and is very close to death.[8]

In Germany, by contrast, the term "euthanasia" is characteristically understood in a way associated with the abuses of the Nazis. In the usual German usage, "euthanasia" has nothing to do with "good death"; it is not a death that is in the interests of the person concerned and preferable to the death the individual might otherwise meet, but is an ostensibly medical procedure performed for ulterior, nonmedical ends. The corruption of the term began first with the concept of "thrift-euthanasia," with the killing of birth-defective infants, and with the infamous T4 program begun at Hitler's direction in 1939, in which chronically ill, retarded, and handicapped Aryans were selected for this "benefit," though many were neither suffering irremediably nor already dying. These programs increasingly moved to the involuntary selection of people, especially mental patients, who were determined unfit for work or who failed other tests of function.[9] The T4 program was discontinued in 1941 as the result of protests from both Protestant and Catholic church leaders, but the personnel from this program were reassigned to the newly opened concentration camps, where they continued to perform killings in the mass exterminations of the Jews, Gypsies, homosexuals, and others regarded as unworthy of life.

With the T4 personnel went not only their technology but the term "euthanasia," and it became firmly associated with Nazi medical experimentation and genocide. In Germany today the term still retains this association with Nazi brutality and the involuntary killing of people for

wholly nonmedical reasons. Indeed, so strong is the stink of the word "euthanasia" in Germany that protest groups have organized to suppress all
discussion of this issue, particularly targeting bioethics lectures and conferences; the mere discussion of euthanasia, these groups have argued,
invites its practice.[10] It is fair to say that the word "euthanasia" can barely
be used in Germany, or indeed in the German language, without arous-
ing concern. While there is some academic discussion of the issue of euthanasia, and while some studies have suggested that the public supports
voluntary active euthanasia (though not called by this label), Germany
as a whole is staunchly opposed to involuntary euthanasia in the sense
associated with the Nazi regime. It relies instead on the practice of assisted suicide, a practice not illegal in Germany, and often employs for
this a distinctive term—"*Freitod*," or "free death"—which has compara-
tively positive connotations.[11]

Thus we can identify two distinct, wholly different senses of the term
"euthanasia," and can note that they are used in these quite opposite ways
in two adjoining European countries. We can call these, loosely, the
"Dutch" and the "German" senses of the term "euthanasia." This is not
simply the distinction between voluntary and involuntary euthanasia,
though of course that distinction is part of it; rather, these terms are
meant to convey the entire connotative range of each of these terms as
they are used in the Netherlands and Germany. Thus "euthanasia" in the
Dutch sense, drawing heavily on the Greek root *euthanatos* or "good
death," means that a patient's life is ended not only at his or her own request but that it is in his or her interests, that it satisfies a set of protec-
tive criteria, that it is buttressed by a set of social supports and acceptance, and that it is essentially free of social stigma. On the other hand,
"euthanasia" in the German sense, evoking the Nazi extermination practices, conveys not only the notion that the killing is involuntary, but that
it is not in the interests of the patient, nor indeed were the interests of
the patient taken into account, that it is motivated by other political or
economic objectives, that it can be brutal in its methods, and that it has
the potential to occur on a very large scale.

When we turn to the United States what we see is that the term "euthanasia" is variously used in ways that approximate both the Dutch and
German senses by various parties in the current debate, and that much
of the dispute is the product of failure to understand the thoroughgoing
equivocation of the term as it is used in both the public and academic

debate. The U.S. debate is neither disciplined by clear definitions of its terms, as in the Netherlands, nor are all the parties to the debate using the term in the already corrupted, post-Nazi sense current in Germany; some use it one way, some use it the other, and because these two senses are not clearly identified as distinct in the public consciousness, many use it shiftingly back and forth.

Consider, as a conveniently self-reflexive example, a passage from comments by Robert D. Orr, M.D.,[12] on an earlier version of this essay (emphases added):

> Professor Battin has clearly presented the traditional arguments for *euthanasia*, namely radical autonomy and compassion, but she has not even attempted to rebut the strongest arguments against physician-performed termination of life. Besides the logical extension to *surrogate voluntary euthanasia* mentioned earlier, there are serious concerns about *euthanasia encouraged or coerced by families;* about *discriminatory euthanasia of the disenfranchised, the disempowered, and the otherwise vulnerable ill.* Then there are the professional concerns about the longstanding absolute prohibition against physicians killing patients; about diversion of efforts from good hospice care; about further erosion of trust between patients and their physicians; and finally about the physician's own conflict of interest (it would often be easier to bend the new rules and kill this patient rather than expend the time, energy, effort, and dollars to care for this severely disabled person). I believe that these arguments are persuasive and that *Graeco-Dutch euthanasia* is too drastic a solution for a few in crisis. I believe there is no place for *euthanasia* as social policy in America's care of its elderly or its terminally ill and it should remain illegal.

In this paragraph, Dr. Orr begins with reference to euthanasia in the Dutch sense; after all, it is for euthanasia in this sense only that I had presented arguments from radical autonomy and compassion. Dr. Orr next speaks of "surrogate voluntary euthanasia," though unless there has been express designation by the patient in an advance directive that another person shall make this choice on his or her behalf, this looks much more simply like one person making a choice about the life of another, and hence is already nonvoluntary and thus outside the orbit of the Dutch sense. Dr. Orr next worries about "euthanasia encouraged or coerced by families." True, a patient's choice of euthanasia might be encouraged by the family and still count as voluntary, but if it is coerced it certainly no longer has anything to do with the Dutch sense of this word and clearly falls far closer to the German sense. The same is true for "discriminatory euthanasia of the disenfranchised, the disempowered and otherwise vulnerable ill": this is precisely what Nazi euthanasia involved. Dr. Orr apparently recognizes that the senses in which he has been using the term "euthanasia" have been shifting, since he begins his conclusion by saying explicitly that "Graeco-Dutch euthanasia is too drastic a solution for a few in crisis"; but he does not seem to notice that his final conclusion, "there is no place for euthanasia as social policy in America's care of its elderly or its terminally ill" is in no way an argument against the view on which he is commenting. What he is actually arguing against is euthanasia in the German sense, not the Dutch one. To make the case he wishes to make here, he would have to advance a slippery-slope argument showing that euthanasia in the Dutch sense inevitably leads to euthanasia in the German sense, but that he does not do; rather, he—like many others in this debate—allows his language to slide around sufficiently to seem to do this work for him. Dr. Orr's concerns are all to be taken seriously, and the prospects of slippery-slope erosion may well be real, but we cannot let shifts in language—in logical terms, a formal equivocation—substitute for careful evidence and real argument.

Thus we can clearly identify two distinct senses of the term "euthanasia," often conflated in discussions of this issue, not only in Dr. Orr's equivocal usage but in much of the academic and public discussion in the United States. To be sure, the actual situation is nowhere near as clear as this; in linguistic reality, there are multiple related senses of the term "euthanasia" approximating the two principal ones I have isolated here. The picture is probably better described as a continuum between two poles, along which various senses of the term in actual usage slide back and forth. Perhaps still better, the picture could be described as a kind of dual Wittgensteinian family of resemblances, with one set of uses forming a "complicated network of similarities overlapping and criss-crossing"[13] around the Dutch sense, and the other— seemingly inextricably intertwined—forming a similar family of interrelated similarities around the German sense. But however the picture of the various senses of the term "euthanasia" might be described, it is clear that there is little consistency, as referents and their associated connotations shift from speaker to speaker and from debate to debate. The result is a generalized failure to communicate. This sort of generalized, thoroughgoing ambiguity and equivocation is far more characteristic of the debate about euthanasia in the United States than it is either in the Netherlands or in Germany. In our arguments about euthanasia, we have to confess, we Americans slide irresponsibly around between the Dutch and the German senses, rarely fully aware of how different these senses really are. As a result, we pay a painful political price for our own lack of conceptual clarity.

Answering the Question(s)

If this is so, then *"Is there a place for euthanasia in America's care for its elderly?"* is not one question, but two. We may pose it in the Dutch sense, and then again, differently, in the post-Nazi sense in which the term is currently understood in Germany; it may invite two quite different answers. Seeing that the question is really two, not one, forces us to recognize that we must be alert to which of the senses is presupposed when a question like the one we set out to consider is asked. Let us, then, consider both possible senses of this question.

Insofar as euthanasia is understood, in the Dutch sense, to be termination of the life of a person at that person's request, and if it is clear that the request is genuine and fully informed, not the product of depression or other emotional or mental disturbance, in an otherwise irremediable medical condition viewed as intolerable by that person, then the answer to the question we have posed would seem simply to be *yes*. If it is what the person earnestly wishes and no other help can be provided to relieve that person's suffering, then it is a form of care that should be provided. But while this *yes* is an answer to the question posed, it also carries with it the presuppositions embedded in the formulation of the question itself. Thus *yes* also requires attention to several further points.

First, although this is a question asked about the elderly, it is not the condition of being elderly that is the basis of one's entitlement to aid-in-dying by means of euthanasia in the Dutch sense; it is suffering an irremediable, usually terminal medical condition that one views as intolerable and for which no acceptable treatment can relieve the suffering. It is one's *medical* condition that first gives rise to a claim on medical assistance; an otherwise healthy person, however elderly, has no claim on medical assistance and no entitlement to medical aid-in-dying, as the terminally ill person does. (This of course has no bearing on the issue of whether an otherwise healthy person, elderly or not, may perform suicide if he or she so chooses.) Thus the question about whether euthanasia in the Dutch sense ought to be made available to the elderly is a question about only some elderly persons, namely those with irremediable, usually terminal medical conditions that they view as intolerable; it is not a question about making physician-performed, medical euthanasia available to all elderly people just because they are old. Furthermore, being elderly is not a prerequisite for "Dutch" euthanasia; if euthanasia is sincerely requested by the person and that person is suffering from an irremediable, probably terminal medical condition for which there is no other acceptable way of relieving suffering, then the age of the person makes little difference, provided only that the individual is adult or old enough, as a mature minor may sometimes be, to count as decisionally competent. To be sure, some elderly persons may wish to bring their lives to an end just because they are elderly, though they do not have other irremediable medical conditions; but this desire, even though it may be quite resolute, does not lay claim on *medical* help in bringing that death about.

Consequently, if "Dutch" euthanasia has a place in America's care for the elderly at all, it is neither for all elderly persons nor confined only to elderly persons. Age is relevant only in that the older person is more likely to be beset with terminal illnesses that cause irremediable suffering, and thus to seek euthanasia. Thus the answer to the question *Is there a place for euthanasia (in the Dutch sense) in America's care for its elderly?* is *yes*, but it is only a subquestion of the larger question *Is there a place for euthanasia (in the Dutch sense) in America's care for its irremediably ill members generally?* To this larger question the answer is also *yes*.

Second, we noted that the question about euthanasia in America's care for its elderly is a question about the provision of care by others, not a question about self-help. This is the case in both medical and financial terms. While I believe that assistance in suicide is also legitimated by the same moral considerations—an appeal to rights of self-determination in matters of one's own dying—as euthanasia in the Dutch sense is legitimated, the argument pursued here is that there should be a place for the social provision of direct aid-in-dying both for those who cannot and those who do not wish to take their own lives. This includes provision of "Dutch" euthanasia for two groups of persons who may wish to turn to it. First are those persons who are prevented by physical handicaps from performing suicide for themselves. No doubt, the most publicly visible such person has been Elizabeth Bouvia, the young California woman rendered virtually completely physically helpless by advanced cerebral palsy and whose petition to a Riverside County court in 1983 to be allowed to starve herself to death attracted national attention. But the second group of persons to whom euthanasia (in the Dutch sense) would be provided is that group of persons physically capable of self-administration of a lethal agent but who prefer to have the procedure performed by someone else. The reasons for this may variously include religious scruples, rooted in traditional prohibitions of suicide; fear of untoward side-effects and incomplete suicide in any attempt at self-administration, resulting in further medical problems; and the wish for the compassionate assistance of a trusted physician, both in providing comfort care for oneself while dying and in providing psychological support for one's family members who may be present during one's dying. While I believe that in the current chaotic and increasingly mercenary health-care situation in the United States assisted suicide provides greater protection against abuse than does physician-performed euthanasia, this is merely a practical rather than theoretical reservation; from a purely moral point of view, the answer to the question of whether there should be a place for euthanasia in the Dutch sense is a resounding *yes*.

But the issue about the provision of such care is not so simple. To claim that euthanasia should be provided is not to say that *only* euthanasia should be provided or that the physician, medical institution, and supporting insurance or other payer is only morally obligated to perform that medical act that brings about death; it also means providing not only this specific service but other related services as well. The actual administration of a lethal agent need not be expensive; but the person requesting euthanasia ought *never* be provided only with this service without access to a further range of services as well, particularly including reconfirmation of diagnoses and prognoses, if requested, treatment for pain and the relief of other symptoms, and the provision of counseling designed not to dissuade but to explore the nature of the request for euthanasia.[14] These latter components, including further diagnostic testing and counseling, can be quite expensive; a society prepared to provide euthanasia in the Dutch sense *must* be prepared to provide these too, without burden to the patient.

This latter point is related to the third presupposition discussed earlier. Euthanasia in the Dutch sense should indeed have a place in America's care for its elderly, but it must actually be "a" place, not the only alternative. It is imperative that reasonable alternatives be available and that they include extensive, humane, guaranteed health care. Otherwise, euthanasia ceases to be an option and becomes the only realistic choice—in which case, it is no longer genuinely a choice at all and cannot be said to be euthanasia in the Dutch sense after all.

Fourth, among the further issues generated by the presuppositions of this issue is the idea of national policy. That there ought to be a place for euthanasia in the Dutch sense in America's care for its elderly does not yet tell us what sort of policy this should be. Directives from agencies like, for example, Health and Human Services or the American Medical Association instructing physicians to perform euthanasia and instructing hospitals and other health care facilities to permit its performance where validly requested by patients are one form of national policy, but not, I believe, the most important one, since these address largely practical matters but do not speak directly to the underlying issue. Rather, it must be recognized that this is an issue of basic civil rights: the rights of individuals to control the circumstances of their own dying. Thus while the question about euthanasia is a question about national policy, not merely local practices, it demands an answer in terms of the most basic civil liberties, not merely bureaucratic dicta. Do Americans have the right to say how they shall die, and whether they may take a route they perceive as easier and more welcome, when they are finally facing death? This issue will no doubt be pursued by advancing aid-in-dying laws in individual states, whether they initially survive or fail the legislative or initiative processes, as for example in Initiative 119, Proposition 161, Measure 16, and proposals emerging in various other states, currently including New Hampshire, Massachusetts, New Mexico, and others. Explicit constitutional challenges to state laws are currently being heard in several federal courts. But while this piecemeal approach may be the only politically realistic strategy, the issue is not properly one under state or local control; it is a basic constitutional issue for all persons.[15]

To say, of course, that the answer to the question *Is there a place for euthanasia (in the Dutch sense) in America's care for its elderly?* should be *yes* is not, of course, to say that there would not be problems with such a practice. The central problem, as many commentators have noted, is to prevent the "slippery slope" slide from voluntary to involuntary euthanasia and hence to moral holocaust—or, in the language of our discussion here, from euthanasia in the Dutch sense to euthanasia in the German one. This was the argument covertly contained in Dr. Orr's equivocal, shifting uses of the term "euthanasia." Whether such a slide would occur, or could be prevented, is the issue to which reflection on both sides of the fence—among both proponents and opponents of legalization—ought to attend.[16]

But as we have seen, the question *Is there a place for euthanasia in America's care for its elderly?* is not just one question, but two, a function of the central ambiguity of the term "euthanasia." The answer to the question in the Dutch sense seems a straightforward *yes.* And the answer to the question in the German sense may seem an even more straightforward *no.* But let us ask it briefly anyway.

If we understand euthanasia in the German sense as killing motivated by quasi-medical or nonmedical considerations, especially including racism and desires for cost control, then euthanasia has no place in America, or anywhere else for that matter. The underlying moral principle justifying (Dutch) euthanasia, as well as physician-assisted suicide at all—the right of the individual to control as far as possible the circumstances of his or her own dying—in no way legitimates euthanasia that is not voluntary, that is not in the interests of the person involved, and that is not performed in the presence of otherwise oncoming death. Furthermore, the various presuppositions of the question as posed are irrelevant here. Whether or not it is limited to the elderly, the practice of involuntary euthanasia in the post-Nazi, German sense is still immoral; whether or not it involves the provision of a "service" by others or relies on self-administration, coerced "aid-in-dying" is still utterly repugnant; whether or not such a policy is national or merely local, it is completely abhorrent in either case; and whether or not there are alternatives is irrelevant: there are no real alternatives if the person can be forced into euthanasia in this way. In short, the answer to the question is a simple, absolute *no,* whatever presuppositions the question may seem to raise.

Thus the answer to the initial question *Is there a place for euthanasia in America's care for its elderly?* may seem to turn out to be quite a simple one after all, a function of recognizing that we usually address this issue in ambiguous ways and that our arguments about it are typically equivocal. When we sort out the distinct senses of "euthanasia" at issue we have no trouble supplying answers for the two different questions that result: *yes,* and *no.*

The Realities of the Situation

But the matter may not be so simple as this easy solution seems to suggest. For if we look carefully at the realities of the situation as they currently are we may see that our practices belie what we say about this issue.

In the United States, which does not currently legally recognize either euthanasia or (except perhaps in Oregon) assisted suicide, the only legally protected option for retaining some degree of control over one's own dying is refusing unwanted treatment, either by withholding new treatment about to be initiated or withdrawing treatment currently in progress. There are three primary mechanisms for exercising one's options to withhold or withdraw treatment: current refusal by a competent patient; an advance directive (either a living will or a durable power of attorney) executed by a patient when competent but that takes effect after the patient becomes incompetent; and determination of the course of treatment to be followed for an incompetent patient by a third party, usually the family or, in disputed cases, the courts. The first two mechanisms, current refusal of treatment by a competent patient, or an advance directive by a patient who was previously competent, appear to trade on the same principle appealed to earlier: the rights of persons to control the circumstances of their own dying—that is, a principle of self-determination. Persons are recognized to have the right to refuse treatment, and they can do so currently or in anticipation of later situations in which they will no longer be competent. But the third mechanism is different. Here, determination by a third party is supplied for the no-longer-competent patient. Though treatments of the third mechanism have been various in the courts, this mechanism attempts to identify what a person's choices would have been in the circumstances at hand, if there is any evidence for doing so—it thus provides "substituted judgment" for that which the person would have made. Only where there is no available evidence or where there cannot be, as in the case of the never-competent patient, does it move to determining what would be in the "best interests" of that person. Thus it is also a mechanism primarily appealing to rights of self-determination, though there are many cases where it cannot do so in practice.

However, the motivation for caring for the elderly is often at odds with this stance of self-determination. The issue is posed in a climate of increasing cost pressures, one in which, it is widely believed, a very substantial portion of health care expenses are devoted to the elderly and those within some months of death. The question, if we are honest about it, arises not only because of concerns about humane care; it is also a question about controlling costs in an out-of-control system. I think it would be seriously wrong to try to disguise this fact from ourselves; on the contrary, I think it is imperative to acknowledge that our concern with the question of euthanasia for the elderly arises from deep uncertainty about the ill state of health care in this country and the fevered costs of medicine. America now has the most expensive health care system in the world, swallowing some 14 percent of the gross domestic product; it is a chaotic system in which efforts to control costs (like the introduction of DRGs, or diagnosis-related groups, as a basis for reimbursement) have not been successful, in which the health status of the populace is declining at the same time costs increase, and in which virtually all parties—including political figures on both sides of the fence, as administrations change—recognize that the system, such as it is, is in grave trouble. Attempts to control costs here in many ways only made things worse.

In this chaotic picture of an inefficient, ineffective system in which costs are out of control, beliefs about the costs of health care for the elderly and the dying play a very large role. Health care for the elderly represents a sizable proportion of total health care costs—after all, virtually the entire Medicare budget is devoted to those over sixty-five. It is also often supposed, though this figure is widely exaggerated, that somewhere around a third of health care costs are spent within the last six months of life (the more accurate figure is probably close to 12–13 percent). These are perceived as very substantial expenses. Furthermore, they are reinforced by perceptions of the high cost of care generally: in the final stages of a terminal illness, hospital care can cost $100,000 a month or more. Since euthanasia is in itself not an expensive procedure and since it precludes further health care costs for any patient to whom it is administered, it is imperative to recognize that the question about euthanasia for the elderly is understood at least in part as a question about whether the overwhelming costs of health care in this country could be controlled by granting *"a place for euthanasia in America's care for its elderly."*

The principal—and most notorious—cost-cutting proposals are those that advocate rationing health care by age. The best known and by far most elegantly presented is Daniel Callahan's, argued originally in his book *Setting Limits: Medical Goals in an Aging Society.*[17] Since there are not enough health care resources or funds to pay for everything for everyone, Callahan and many others argue, health care must be rationed, and the just basis on which to ration is age. Thus health care would go to the young; the elderly would have the last priority for receiving care. According to these proposals for age rationing, this ranking of priorities—young first, elderly last—is justified because (though different proposals explicate the matter in slightly different ways) the elderly have already lived a normal life span; in remaining alive, they have already benefited from whatever health care they may have needed. To give full care to the elderly, in a scarcity situation, would be to deprive some of the young of care necessary to continue their lives, and they would die before reaching the normal life span; to give full care to the young, on the other hand, might deprive the elderly of care they also need to continue their lives—but the lives of the elderly have already continued to the point where they have had a fair share of life.

This argument is often pursued on underlying Rawlsian grounds, mediated by the detailed application to health care provided by Norman Daniels.[18] Daniels argues that Rawls's rational self-interest maximizers in the Original Position, agreeing to principles of justice from behind the veil of ignorance in which they do not know their own individual characteristics (including their own health statuses and likely causes of death), would in a condition of scarcity select an age-rationing principle for the distribution of health care. This is because providing more efficient health care earlier in life, at a time prerequisite to living at all later on, would increase the prospects of reaching a normal life span for all. I do not think the age-rationing principle is unjust; on the contrary, were the situation one of genuine (rather than bureaucratically, institutionally engendered) scarcity, and were it occurring in a world characterized by just institutions, I would think the theoretical conclusion right, that priority in care should go to the young rather than the elderly. But the practical conclusion almost universally drawn in the United States from this theoretical stance, that age rationing here and now is therefore justified, does not automatically follow. This has not only to do with the fact that our scarcity is not clearly genuine and that our background institutions are not just, but also to do with the fact that age rationing is not voluntary. Hence age rationing is in conflict with the underlying principle that persons have the right to self-determination in matters of their own dying. This principle cannot be overridden if there are other alternatives that can achieve both a practical distribution of resources in accord with the demands of justice and yet preserve voluntary choice. The solution, it seems to me,[19] is to assure both full health care for the elderly *and* euthanasia—but euthanasia *only in the Dutch sense*. It must be euthanasia that is *fully* voluntary, not coerced either by the lack of humane alternatives or by any bureaucratic policy. The assumption that underlies this view is that given a genuinely open choice between, on the one hand, "Dutch" euthanasia and its near relative, assisted suicide, and on the other hand continuing treatment, the savings realized by those who choose euthanasia or some form of aid-in-dying will be extensive enough to fund full care for those who choose to press on.

This is of course a rebuttable presumption. It is not very well supported by current data from the Netherlands, where, the Remmelink Commission has found, only 1.8 percent of patients dying in a given year choose euthanasia and only an additional 0.3 percent choose physician-assisted suicide.[20] To be sure, in some areas the figures are different: some 10 to 15 percent of all AIDS patients in the Netherlands choose euthanasia. But these are figures from a society in which euthanasia is only beginning to be accepted—within the last twenty years—and is still technically illegal. In 1990, reporting procedures under Dutch law were modified to offer a physician greater protection from prosecution if euthanasia is performed according to a strict set of guidelines, even though euthanasia remains illegal; it is already evident that this additional protection has increased Dutch physicians' willingness to report. What is not clear is whether it has also increased Dutch physicians' actual willingness to assist patients in dying—though the vast majority say they are prepared to do so—and whether, were rights to aid-in-dying by euthanasia or assisted suicide still more fully assured among one's other civil rights and liberties, it will also increase the frequency with which patients make such choices.

Robert Kastenbaum suggests that a day may come in which practices of suicide will become "the preferred mode of death" because they allow a person control over the time, place, duration, immediate cause, and style of dying.[21] One can easily imagine the development of religious rites surrounding such choices, patterns of familial comfort and involvement, and many other factors that would increase the attractiveness of a self-directed death in preference to a medically dictated one. Since some 70 to 80 percent of all persons in the technologically advanced nations can expect to

die of deteriorative conditions typically marked by long downhill cours-
es late in life, if a substantial proportion of persons facing such ends were
to choose as Kastenbaum predicts they eventually will, such choices would
indeed solve the distributive problem of allocation of health care to the
elderly—but *not* by involuntary imposition or disenfranchisement from
care. Whether Kastenbaum's prediction will come true we of course cannot say, but we can already see what would be important about it: this,
compared to any alternative scheme for coping with distributive scarcity,
best protects the fundamental principle of autonomy in matters of one's
own dying. It is this principle that is central; it both speaks for the recognition of euthanasia in the Dutch sense and against recognition of euthanasia in the German one. If dying patients do not voluntarily make
such choices in a way sufficient to offset the cost pressures society is experiencing, some other way must be found to resolve the distributive issue—but not by coercive, involuntary euthanasia—that is, euthanasia in
the German sense.

But it also points out in what ways the strategies we are beginning to
employ for controlling costs—involuntary rationing—more strongly resemble the latter than the former, and it is here that the fifth of our earlier presuppositions about the question concerning euthanasia arises—the assumption that active and passive euthanasia are two distinct phenomena, and
that we can explore the issue of one without scrutinizing the other. Let us
look more closely at the strategies we already have in place for protecting
patient choice—and, in the bargain, controlling costs.

We already have legally recognized structures for persons who wish to
stipulate their wishes about care after they are no longer competent: the
Living Will and the Durable Power of Attorney. But we do not rigorous-
ly honor these choices. In a 1991 study of advance directives for life-sustaining care among nursing home patients, care was consistent with the
previously expressed wishes of the patient only 75 percent of the time;
and of the patients whose care was inconsistent with their expressed wishes, 25 percent got more aggressive treatment, while 75 percent had treatment withheld though they did not request this.[22] Of course, ignoring
patients' wishes does not always mean that care they might have wanted
is denied them; often patients get care they do not want. A study published early in 1993 revealed that doctors and nurses—some 1,400 at five
major medical centers were surveyed—say they often violate their own

personal beliefs and ignore requests from patients to withhold life support in cases of terminal illness.[23] Almost 50 percent of attending physicians and nurses and 70 percent of resident physicians reported acting
against their conscience in overtreating terminally ill patients, even when
there was no chance for recovery and death was considered imminent.
Four times as many of those surveyed were concerned about overtreat-
ment as were concerned about undertreatment of dying patients. These
doctors and nurses were often unaware of national directives and hospital policies that permit withdrawal of treatment, but they also said they
were dissatisfied with the way patients were involved in treatment decisions. The *New York Times* rapidly pointed out that in ignoring patients'
desires, medical personnel may also be "substantially contributing to the
uncontrolled escalation of health care costs."[24]

What is essential here is not just whether patients are being overtreated or undertreated, as these studies seem to suggest, but the prevalence
of ignoring patients' wishes. Furthermore, it appears that patients' wishes are not ignored primarily for reasons of their—the patients'—interests but for a variety of extrinsic, institutional, legal, or custom-driven
reasons instead. While there may be vast differences in outcome for the
patient who is overtreated from the one who is undertreated, both patients suffer the same offense: namely, their wishes are ignored. Nor is
there any reason to think that if the wishes of terminally ill patients are
ignored, the wishes of elderly patients will not be ignored as well.

To be sure, there is new legislation designed to reinforce patient choice.
The Patient Self-Determination Act, effective December 1, 1991, requires
that hospitalized or institutionalized patients be asked if they have advance
directives—and many such patients will have been urged in these circumstances to execute them. But even legislation such as this cannot guarantee
reflective choice, the product of sustained, profound consideration. For one
thing, these choices to withhold or withdraw treatment are likely to be elic-
ited in circumstances that are potentially coercive—namely, at the time of
admission to a hospital, often an urgent, frightening time—and so may not
reflect genuine choice. Furthermore, even without pressure or coercion,
there is evidence that patients often do not understand the effect of the
advance directives they are executing. In a 1991 study of whether hospitalized patients with and without advance directives actually understood the
force and content of them, those who had actually signed advance direc-

tives performed almost as poorly on tests of comprehension of these directives as those who did not have them: these patients with advance directives did not know what the directives covered, in what circumstances they applied, or what forms of treatment they would permit or prohibit.[25] In addition, the range of choices open to a patient is artificially limited: the advance directive permits choices of withholding or withdrawing treatment, but not choices of euthanasia or suicide. Thus what seems to be a choice is only a partial choice, and one that may seem to be neither fully informed nor fully voluntary. Not fully voluntary, not fully informed withdrawing or withholding of treatment may seem a long way from the wholly involuntary killings of the Nazi form of euthanasia, but it still shares some features with it: death is brought about without the understanding, request, or consent of the patient.

These are, of course, all cases of passive euthanasia, not the active sort we began by addressing. But if we challenge the presupposition of our initial question, that we can regard active and passive euthanasia as distinct, we must raise the issue of whether our behavior with respect to passive euthanasia does not have some bearing on our behavior with respect to active euthanasia as well. Does what we say and what we do in passive euthanasia tell us something about what we might say and do in active euthanasia as well? The practice we rely on for responding to cost pressures— passive euthanasia by withholding and withdrawing treatment—does not emphasize self-determination, and it proposes a solution to the distributive problem not by enhancing but by restricting choice. Of course, we often do not practice withholding and withdrawing treatment in a coherent way, and we often overtreat rather than undertreat, but when we do we deplore the cost consequences of our actions.

Thus we can ask one last time, *Is there a place for euthanasia in America's care for its elderly?* The answer is *yes* if we are speaking of euthanasia in the Dutch sense; the answer is *no,* if by this we have euthanasia in the German sense in mind. The former ought not be regarded as merely a policy option: it is a matter of right; while the latter is repugnant on all counts and ought be permitted in no way. Yet we note widespread erosion of the principle of voluntary choice, that central feature that is the basis of the differentiation between "Dutch" and "German" euthanasia, of the forms we should accept and reject. To be sure, the principle of voluntary choice cannot always be preserved in situations of extreme scarcity; these are issues of whom is to be thrown from the lifeboat. But ours is a situation of mild to moderate scarcity, much of which is occasioned by institutional inefficiency and misplaced priorities in the health care system. Thus we are faced with a practical dilemma, just as our conceptual confusion is resolved. While we see that euthanasia in the benign sense might both increase patients' range of choices and at the same time relieve distributive pressures that seem to speak for the restriction of choice in the first place, yet we cannot promote euthanasia for reasons of cost control, for this is to slide already into that repugnant form of euthanasia we ought most urgently to avoid. *Is there a place for euthanasia in America's care for its elderly?* Yes, in the Dutch sense. No, in the post-Nazi sense. The trick is to get one for America's elderly without also getting the other.

Notes

1. The question was originally framed this way by James Walters and Duane Covrig, organizers of the conference "Rationing Health Care: Ethics and Aging," at the Center for Christian Bioethics, Loma Linda University, March 1–2, 1992, at which this essay was first presented. I thank them for comments on an earlier draft.

2. See Margaret P. Battin, *The Least Worst Death: Essays in Bioethics on the End of Life* (New York: Oxford University Press, 1994), 130–44, a portion of which appeared as "Seven Caveats concerning the Discussion of Euthanasia in Holland" in *Perspectives in Biology and Medicine* 34:1 (1990): 73–77.

3. See, for example, the recommendations by Timothy E. Quill, M.D., Christine K. Cassel, M.D., and Diane E. Meier, M.D., "Care of the Hopelessly Ill: Proposed Clinical Criteria for Physician-Assisted Suicide," *New England Journal of Medicine* 327:19 (1992): 1380–83. The recommendations follow the Dutch guidelines fairly closely, though they are not identical.

4. Most recent proposals in the United States have concerned only physician-assisted suicide and would not legalize physician-performed euthanasia. However, because of the relevance of the linguistic issues concerning the ambiguous meanings of the term "euthanasia" for the debate in the United States, I will be considering both.

5. P. van der Maas, J. van Delden, L. Pijnenborg, and C. Looman, "Euthanasia and Other Medical Decisions concerning the End of Life," *The Lancet* 338 (Sept. 14, 1991): 669–74. This study is known as the Remmelink Commission Report; the full text is available in English as a special issue of *Health Policy* 22:1–2 (1992). See also G. van der Wal, J. Th. M. Van Eijk, H. J. J. Leenen, and C. Spreeuwenberg, "Euthanasie en hulp bij selfdoding door artsen in de thuissituatie," *Ned Tijdschr Geneeskd* 135:35 (1991).

6. Remmelink Commission Report, 609.

7. Ibid., 672.

8. The LAWER cases (which total about 0.8 percent of total annual deaths, while euthanasia cases total 1.8 percent and physician-assisted suicide cases total 0.3 percent) are examined in Loes Pijnenborg, Paul J. van der Maas, Johannes J. M. van Delden, and Caspar W. N. Looman, "Life-Terminating Acts without Explicit Request of Patient," *The Lancet* 341 (May 8, 1993): 1196–99. This study finds just two cases, both from the early 1980s, in which a competent patient was euthanized without that patient's knowledge.

9. For an account of these programs, see Robert Jay Lifton, *The Nazi Doctors: Medical Killing and the Psychology of Genocide* (New York: Basic Books, 1986), especially part 1.

10. See Bettina Schöne-Seifert and Klaus-Peter Rippe, "Silencing the Singer: Antibioethics in Germany," *Hastings Center Report* 21:6 (1991): 20–27. Some recent observers suggest this opposition is quieting down.

11. See Margaret P. Battin, "Assisted Suicide: Can We Learn from Germany?" *Hastings Center Report* 22:2 (1992): 44–51, which also appears in Battin, *Least Worst Death*, 254–70.

12. Unpublished manuscript, courtesy of the author, from the conference at which this essay was originally presented.

13. Ludwig Wittgenstein, *Philosophical Investigations* (New York: Macmillan, 1958), paragraph I:66, p. 32ᵉ.

14. For concrete suggestions about counseling in such situations, see Margaret P. Battin, "Rational Suicide? How Can We Respond to a Request for Help?" *Crisis (Journal of the International Association for Suicide Prevention)* 12:2 (1991): 73–80, which also appears in Battin, *Least Worst Death*, 271–76.

15. See Alan L. Sullivan, "A Constitutional Right to Suicide," in M. Pabst Battin and David J. Mayo, eds., *Suicide: The Philosophical Issues* (New York: St. Martin's Press, 1980), 229–53.

16. See Margaret P. Battin, "Voluntary Euthanasia and the Risks of Abuse: Can We Learn Anything from the Netherlands?" *Law, Medicine, and Health Care* 20:1 (1992): 133–43, which also appears in Battin, *Least Worth Death*, 163–81.

17. Daniel Callahan, *Setting Limits: Medical Goals in an Aging Society* (New York: Simon and Schuster, 1987).

18. Norman Daniels, *Am I My Parents' Keeper? An Essay on Justice between the Young and the Old* (New York: Oxford University Press, 1988), and later works (see chap. 2 in this volume).

19. See Margaret P. Battin, "Age-Rationing and the Just Distribution of Health Care: Is There a Duty to Die?" *Ethics* 97:2 (1987): 317–40, which also appears in Battin, *Least Worst Death*, 58–79.

20. Van der Maas et al., "Euthanasia and Other Medical Decisions," 671.

21. Robert Kastenbaum, "Suicide as the Preferred Way of Death," in Edwin S. Shneidman, ed., *Suicidology: Contemporary Developments* (New York: Grune and Stratton, 1976), 425–41.

22. Marion Danis, M.D., et al., "A Prospective Study of Advance Directives for Life-Sustaining Care," *New England Journal of Medicine* 324:13 (1991): 882–88. The authors recognize that their study was of a small population and that further empirical research is necessary to generalize their findings.

23. Mildred Solomon et al., "Decisions Near the End of Life: Professional Views on Life-Sustaining Treatment," *American Journal of Public Health* 83:1 (1993): 14–23.

24. Jane E. Brody, "Doctors Admit Ignoring Dying Patients' Wishes," *New York Times*, Jan. 14, 1993, A-12.

25. Jay A. Jacobson, M.D., Barbara E. White, Margaret P. Battin, Ph.D., Leslie P. Francis, Ph.D., J.D., David Green, M.D., and Evelyn S. Kasworm, "Patients' Understanding and Use of Advance Directives," *Western Journal of Medicine* 160:3 (1994): 232–36.

4

Caring for the Disabled Elderly
The Economics and Ethics of Financing Long-Term Care

Nancy S. Jecker

Since the 1980s the specter of rationing lifesaving and life-prolonging health care on the basis of age has sparked debate among health professionals and in the wider community.[1] Debate has centered on assessing the value of extending life once persons have passed the marker of a "natural life span." Although life-extension in old age is an important concern, this essay emphasizes that the overwhelming health needs of older Americans are not for dramatic, lifesaving interventions. Rather, older individuals need ongoing treatment for chronic disabling conditions and mundane assistance with activities of daily living. Thus the greater challenge for society in the next century will not be to ensure the availability of acute, high technology medicine for the nation's elderly, but to invest in care-oriented, low technology health care services for older adults. While hospitals will have increasing trouble filling their beds, more nursing homes will need to be constructed to accommodate the increasing ranks of chronically disabled elderly. According to one estimate, there will be two to three times as many individuals aged eighty-five and over in nursing homes in the year 2040 as there are individuals aged sixty-five and over in nursing homes today.[2]

It is somewhat ironic therefore that so much attention has been paid to the prospect of disenfranchising the elderly from life-extending interventions, while the entrenched practice of failing to protect individuals against the catastrophic costs of long-term care is hardly mentioned. Moreover, although rationing of health care of any sort to the elderly disproportionately affects women, because of the greater numbers of older women,[3] it is older men who have, on average, relatively greater needs for acute care interventions. Thus, the present debate about whether or not to redirect lifesaving resources from the old to the young focuses the discussion of elder care on health services used primarily by older men. The absence of debate about chronic disability and coverage for long-term care glosses over an area of health care that is especially vital to the well being of older women.

This essay first describes the public financing of long-term care through Medicaid and Medicare and draws out the implications of this analysis. I show that one effect of limiting reimbursement for long-term care is that society indirectly rations health care on the twin bases of age and gender. The second section of the essay puts forth an argument to show that justice mandates allocating a substantially larger share of public monies to long-term care. I claim that long-term care merits priority because ongoing assistance with activities of daily living is a prerequisite to self-respect for the functionally disabled. The final part of the essay explores public versus private financing of long-term care. I argue that private resources to pay for long-term care are likely to remain inadequate.

The Public Financing of Long-Term Care

In the United States we invest relatively few public resources in supportive services and long-term care for chronic disabling conditions. Long-term care includes services such as adult day care, in-home services and care in resident facilities, convalescent homes, and intermediate and skilled nursing facilities. Such services are needed as a result of chronic disabilities caused by diseases such as Alzheimer's, osteoporosis, heart disease, or stroke. Rather than devoting resources to these "low technology" services, we choose to devote the majority of society's health care dollars to acute care medicine, largely in the form of intensive, short-term, hospital care that is crisis-driven. Medicaid, the federal- and state-financed entitlement program designed to meet the health care needs of low-income individuals, makes home health care a mandatory benefit. Despite this, Medicaid contributes less than 2 percent of its budget nationally to home care services.[4] While states are allowed under Medicaid to offer acute home-based care, personal care that includes assistance with personal needs, and waiver programs aimed at keeping people in the community, only half of states offer coverage for these services. States have a strong incentive under Medicaid to limit all forms of home services because they cannot be limited to a pre-budgeted amount, but instead must be offered to all recipients.

Medicaid pays a substantially greater portion of the cost of nursing home care for the indigent, with two-fifths of all Medicaid payments going to nursing homes.[5] Elderly persons with Medicaid coverage who need nursing home care receive assistance with Medicare premiums and cost sharing, as well as coverage for additional benefits. Yet coverage under Medicaid is uneven between states and eligibility requirements fall below federal poverty guidelines in many states. Thus, a majority (60 percent) of the poor are not covered by Medicaid. The limited reach of Medicaid means that less than one-third of disabled elderly receive Medicaid assistance.[6] The fact that eligibility for Medicaid is means-tested also means that ill and disabled elderly people must substantially reduce assets and savings they may have accumulated over a lifetime to become eligible. Thus spouses may be compelled to divorce their life-long partners to protect their assets. Among the current nursing home population covered by Medicaid, approximately 50 percent were initially private-pay patients who significantly spent down their personal financial resources to pay for nursing home costs before receiving Medicaid.[7]

Since its inception in 1965, Medicare, the nation's primary form of health insurance for the elderly, has also emphasized coverage for acute and life-threatening medical problems, rather than chronic disabling conditions. In 1985, less than 1 percent of Medicare expenditures went to nursing home care.[8] Medicare pays primarily out-of-hospital costs associated with short term, post-acute illness care. In this area, Medicare pays only for skilled nursing care needed after discharge from a hospital, and then only for twenty days of nursing home care and assistance with the cost of eighty additional days. Despite these limits, the need for nursing home care has increased dramatically since the introduction of prospective payment for Medicare hospital patients.[9] Hospitals have shortened the length of hospital stays for patients and discharged them "quicker and sicker."

In the area of home health care, Medicare represents the primary formal funding source, yet home health care comprises only 3 percent of overall Medicare costs.[10] As a result of the limited nature of Medicare coverage, most (70 percent) severely impaired elderly people living in the community receive no paid assistance, and a quarter of total spending on in-home services for the elderly is paid out of pocket.[11]

Impact on Elderly Women

Limited access to long-term care impacts the elderly population disproportionately because the successful application of modern technology to
what were once fatal conditions has prolonged lives and increased the
duration of many chronic disabling conditions.[12] Thus the elderly are
more likely than other age groups to experience chronic illness and functional disability. Persons over sixty-five are 4.5 times more likely to experience activity limitation than persons who are younger than sixty-
five.[13]

Rationing that befalls the elderly disproportionately also affects more
women than men, because women are disproportionately represented
among older adults. On average, women outlive men by 7.5 years.[14] In
the group aged sixty-five and over, there are sixty-eight men per one hundred women; for ages eighty-five and over, forty-five men per one hundred women.[15] The explanation for these sex differences is that at birth,
each birth cohort includes slightly greater numbers of men than women.
However, men's mortality rates are higher than women's at all ages, so
the number of women in each birth cohort eventually equals and then
surpasses the number of men.

In addition to the sheer number of older women, older women are disproportionately represented among older nursing home and home health
care clientele. Among the 1.2 million elderly residents of nursing homes,
almost 75 percent are women,[16] and about 65 percent of elderly persons
needing home care are women.[17] These statistics reflect the fact that older men are more likely than older women to be afflicted by diseases that
lead to death. At ages sixty-five to sixty-nine, men die at twice the rate of
women.[18] Thus the list of medical conditions with higher rates for older
men contains many of the leading causes of death for persons over sixty-five, such as heart disease, cerebrovascular disease, arteriosclerosis,
pneumonia, emphysema/asthma.[19] By contrast, older women are more
likely than older men to suffer from multiple chronic conditions that are
not life-threatening; older women are also more likely to experience
difficulty in performing social, physical, and mobility activities.[20] For example, older women's rates are higher for hypertension, arthritis, diabe-
tes, anemia, migraine, sciatica, hypertensive disease, varicose veins, most
digestive problems, allergies, and most orthopedic problems.[21] These conditions are frequently symptomatic, but infrequently fatal.

As a consequence of these sex differences, older men make greater use of hospitals, which Medicare reimburses, whereas older women use more prescription medicine and utilize more custodial services in homes and institutions, for which Medicare provides no or little reimbursement.[22] The result is that Medicare covers a smaller portion of older women's health care needs than older men's. In 1986, for example, Medicare paid 49 percent of the total health care costs for unmarried men over sixty-five, 44 percent for older married couples, but only 33 percent of health care costs for unmarried older women.[23]

Since elderly women experience poverty at higher rates than their male counterparts,[24] they are also more financially burdened by the cost of paying for uncovered health care. Women over sixty-five constitute the single poorest group in the country, with one third falling below the federal poverty level.[25] Because few of them worked outside the home, today's elderly women receive less from Social Security or private pension benefits than their male peers. Thus although women constitute 58.7 percent of persons sixty-five and over, they account for 72.4 percent of all elderly people beneath the poverty level.[26] Widowed or never-married women over eighty have the highest risk of needing in-home or nursing home care, but the average annual income in this group is less than $6,000.[27]

A final reason why limiting access to long-term care is especially onerous for older women is that functional impairments have the potential to disrupt more significantly the lives of older women. On the one hand, older women are far more likely than older men to be divorced, never married or widowed, and so less likely to have a spouse on whom to rely.[28] On the other hand, even among married persons living with their spouses, functional impairments may impact the daily activities of older women more. Today's older women belong to a cohort of women who have assumed primary responsibility for domestic tasks, such as cooking, shopping, and house cleaning. When chronic disability interferes with their capacity to carry out these activities, they may be less able than older men to continue life as usual by relying on their spouse.[29]

The Impending Crisis

Having considered the implications of emphasizing acute high technology services over chronic low technology assistance, we need next to explore more directly the problems of rationing and equitable distribution of health care this raises. Although rationing of long-term care is already with us, in the years ahead it will be far more pervasive. For a variety of reasons, the need for long-term care is expected to increase well into the twenty-first century. Between 1980 and 2000, the United States population is expected to grow 18 percent and the need for long-term care will increase 38 percent. Between 2000 and 2040, the nation's population is projected to grow 20 percent and the number of people needing extensive long-term care may swell by as much as 60 percent.[30]

One factor that will contribute to the greater demand for long-term care is that the ratio of older women to older men will widen. Although women are already disproportionately present in older age groups, the sex differential in life expectancy is expected to increase until the year 2050, at which time it will level off. But before it does, there will be only 38.8 men per one hundred women age eighty-five and over. By 2050, life expectancy for women will be 81 and for men 71.8 years, a 9.2 year difference.[31] As suggested already, the significance of these figures is that older women experience a greater incidence of morbidity and disability than older men. Thus when more older people are women, the need for long-term care will be correspondingly greater.

A second factor that will lead to a greater need for long-term care is the burgeoning of the aged population over eighty-five. This group constitutes the fastest growing portion of the population. Since 1900, those over the age of eighty-five have become twenty-one times as numerous,[32] and between 1960 and 1980 alone the population of Americans eighty-five and over increased by 141 percent. Demographers predict that future trends will continue to reflect a surge in growth of extremely old people. Further, a growing number of individuals in the oldest age group will be one hundred or more years old. The population of U.S. centenarians is forecast to increase from 15,000 in 1980 to 110,000 by the year 2000; by the year 2050, the number of Americans over 100 years old will be as high as 300,000 to 500,000.[33]

What makes these figures relevant is that the oldest old are the heaviest users of long-term care. More than 70 percent of those eighty-five and over require some kind of assistance with one or more activities of daily living.[34] Among the relatively healthier noninstitutionalized elderly, 36 percent of persons eighty-five and over have one or more limitations in activities of daily living.[35] These figures are significantly greater than corresponding figures for the "young old." For example, whereas 20 percent of those over sixty-five have multiple disease processes that limit normal activity, after the age of eighty-five 46 percent of those living in the community experience such limitations.[36] In the foreseeable future the steep rise in chronic disease and disability associated with very old age is unlikely to change.[37] There is, for example, little evidence to suggest that a compression of morbidity will occur, with life expectancy leveling off around age eighty-five or ninety, and the period of time spent in chronic illness and disability declining.[38]

Third, the crisis in long-term care is expected to worsen because fewer offspring will be available to provide informal care for the future generation of elderly. Already, the average married couple has more parents than children.[39] During the 1990s the total number of births will drop, but the population over sixty-five will increase.[40] This imbalance between the population of young and the population of old will place greater strain on families because fewer children will be available to share the emotional and financial costs of caregiving. In addition, women, who make up the vast majority of family caregivers, are entering the paid labor force in growing numbers. Fewer than one in ten families conform to the traditional model of one parent at home while the other parent works. During the next decade, almost two thirds of new employees will be women.[41]

Ethical Values Supporting Long-Term Care

Having established that there will be a tremendous need for long-term care services, let us next consider the ethical questions this raises. First, how should a humane society respond in the face of this immense and growing need for long-term care? Second, on what bases might an ethic of responsibility be founded?

It might at first glance be thought that the importance of investing in services that assist people with mundane activities of daily living pales in significance when compared to other resource priorities, such as life-saving or life-prolonging treatment. Yet problems of everyday living, when added together, determine the overall quality of individuals' lives.[42] How such problems are dealt with ultimately affects whether individuals retain autonomy and dignity at the end of life.

Yet what, more specifically, gives ethical urgency to the frail elderly's need for assistance with bathing, toileting, dressing, and moving about? Why should helping the disabled deal with the nagging indignities of daily life be regarded as a resource priority? One answer to this question is that caring for the elderly disabled in these ways is necessary to protect their self-determination and self-respect. Self-respect refers to a person's sense of his or her own value, and it implies a confidence in one's ability, so far as possible, to realize one's goals and values.[43] Self-respect erodes when persons are led to doubt persistently their own worth or are frustrated repeatedly in their attempts to carry out their plans.[44]

An individual's capacity to develop and sustain self-respect also depends crucially upon receiving the respect of others. For example, self-respect is hindered when society signals unequal respect for persons by providing unequal access to goods that are essential to security and opportunities.[45] For the disabled elderly, self-respect can become imperiled when assistance getting out of bed, moving about, and eating is not available. The paucity of social resources devoted to providing such assistance conveys that disabled elderly individuals are not a valued presence in society and are not granted equal standing with others. From the perspective of the disabled elderly person, such a message may encourage the erroneous belief that one's rightful place in a moral community is below others. In other words, those who find their needs ignored or denigrated by others may abjectly accept these responses as truly deserved. One reason that such a self-perception may arise is that "Most people hate to think of themselves as victims . . . [and] would rather reorder reality than admit that [they] are the helpless objects of injustice."[46]

Believing that one is fundamentally inferior, in turn, elicits feelings of shame and self-hatred. Aristotle describes shame as "a kind of fear of dishonor" that "produces an effect similar to that produced by fear of danger."[47] According to Aristotle, it is particularly wounding to fear dishonor and feel shame in old age, because honor is especially due the elderly individual. It is especially fitting to recognize that by old age persons have accomplished the considerable feat of meeting the multiple challenges of living. As Albert Jonsen puts it, "Living a life is an achievement. Some persons do it with great vigor and style; others barely make it; yet everyone who survives accomplishes it. The accomplishment deserves acknowledgment."[48]

In addition to requiring the respect of others, having a sure sense of one's own worth requires some degree of success in carrying out the plans and goals one sets. For example, functional impairments such as vision, hearing, or speech deficits have the potential to impede self-respect and self-esteem because they prevent people from executing even the most ordinary and modest goals, such as talking on the telephone or reading a newspaper. Services compensating for sensory impairments facilitate feelings of self worth by enabling self-confidence to develop about one's ability to perform tasks and realize goals.

It is important to understand that the erosion of self-respect that can accompany chronic disabilities has a cumulative effect. Although a single incident of bladder or bowel incontinence, or a single event of difficulty getting in and out of a chair, does not irreparably damage a person's self-esteem, repeated episodes are harder to ignore or write off. Over time, an accumulated history of failures can "teach" persons to feel helpless. Moreover, when helplessness is learned with respect to a specific task, it is easily generalized to other circumstances. When this occurs, individuals come to believe they are helpless in areas where they have no history of performance failure.[49] In the case of the disabled elderly person, an insidious process can be set in motion whereby events that are within one's power are viewed as response independent or "beyond one's control." In this way, recurrent failure at performing seemingly trivial tasks has the potential to weaken dramatically a person's sense of self-worth and to reduce significantly a person's physical and emotional security and life chances.

Persons who have experienced a gradual loss of self-confidence and self-respect over time are also less prepared to fend off further assaults on personal dignity. In this sense, the current program for financing long-term care through Medicaid serves the disabled especially poorly. As noted already, eligibility for Medicaid requires disabled people to reduce substantially any assets and savings they have accumulated over a lifetime. The process of relinquishing personal assets and beggaring health care is undeniably a demeaning and degrading experience. On the one hand, for many people self-esteem is inextricably linked to possessions and to the lifestyle patterns with which possessions are associated. When individuals are forcibly cut loose from long-standing ways of living, the sense of identity built around these lifestyle habits begins to falter. On the other hand, even individuals who are already near poverty and must give up relatively little to qualify for Medicaid may be deeply affected by spending down. Those who live on the edge of poverty can come to cherish their assets more because they are fewer, and they can reasonably feel panic about what others regard as relatively minor financial losses.

The requirement to reduce personal resources also hinders self-respect by interrupting the family ritual of passing wealth from one generation to the next. For some, this ritual may be a source of enormous pride and a symbol of family solidarity. The execution of a will and the naming of one's inheritors can convey an elderly individual's authority and power to family members at a time when the elder's sense of authority and power are otherwise waning. Thus control over family wealth can bolster the elderly person's sense of self-esteem and standing relative to younger generations.

Taken together, these points about self-respect and self-determination suggest an ethical framework for thinking about the priority that long-term care merits in the overall health care scheme. First, guaranteeing access to long-term care on the basis of health care needs conveys that persons with disabilities have equal worth and dignity. This in turn supports self-determination and self-respect for disabled persons. By contrast, requiring that disabled individuals become impoverished in order to qualify for long-term care merely adds insult to injury. The impoverishment requirement erodes further the already imperiled value of personal dignity. Although society cannot apportion self-respect and dignity among its members, it can distribute the conditions that make it possible to attain these goods.

Second, financing long-term care and promoting conditions of self-respect is a concern of justice. Long-term care gains ethical urgency not simply because we should act compassionately to promote the good of persons, but rather because the conditions that make self-respect possible are something to which people are entitled.[50] This is because justice transcends the problem of allocating specific material resources and incorporates broader issues involving the distribution of liberties, powers, and opportunities. Justice, in its traditional formulation in Western culture, refers not only to the allocation of material property but also to "complete virtue in its fullest sense," including the awarding of honor and dishonor. Just action in this sense corresponds to actions prescribed under "rightly-framed law" and "we call those acts just that tend to produce and preserve happiness and its components for the political society."[51] As others have noted, laws and social institutions that compensate individuals for the contingencies of nature and social circumstance enable human flourishing because the public affirmation of each person's endeavors supports their self-esteem.[52] Although the loss of physical prowess that can accompany aging is not itself remediable, it is possible to compensate for these losses and make possible an honorable and decent old age.

Finally, within justice debates, long-term care merits priority because over time it profoundly affects the quality of life individuals lead. While saving and extending life is an important value, the quality of life to be achieved is a concern of equal weight. Just as few would wish to be rescued from death only to live a wretched life, so few would intentionally choose a health care system that saves lives but lacks the resources necessary to make possible a worthwhile and dignified life.

Public versus Private Responsibility

Translating these values into reform of the nation's financing of long-term care is the challenge that lies ahead. A central question that reforms must address is, Where do the duties of individuals and families end, and society's responsibilities begin? In particular, How should the financial responsibility of supporting dependent elderly people be shared by different groups in society? As noted already, today in the United States disabled elderly persons who use long-term care generally pay for it out of pocket or turn to welfare. Comparisons between the financing of acute hospital-based services versus long-term care provide a useful vantage point. In the area of long-term care, over 50 percent is financed by the elderly and their families as out of pocket expenses; 40 percent by state and federal tax revenues used to fund the Medicaid program; 5 percent through social security taxes used for Medicare; and 5 percent from miscellaneous sources, including just over 1 percent from private long-term care insurance.[53] By contrast, less than 10 percent of hospital expenditures come directly from patients, and over 90 percent are paid through private and social insurance mechanisms.[54] It is not clear what the justification is for this discrepancy. For example, why should a middle-income elderly individual needing long-term care in a nursing home be subject to a means-tested program that requires reducing assets and income substantially to become eligible, while the same individual's hospital services are routinely paid for by public insurance? In 1993 (following passage of the Omnibus Reconciliation Act of 1993), a couple with assets of $150,000 would be required (in most states) to spend half of their assets before becoming eligible to receive Medicaid. If the same couple had devoted money to a child's college education, or assisted with a son's or daughter's mortgage payment, they would not be eligible for Medicaid for three years after the date these assets were dispersed. If the couple had transferred funds to a trust, the waiting period would be five years.

To allow the current imbalance between public financing of acute versus long-term care to continue would be unethical. One reason for making this judgment focuses on the character and values that such a bias perpetuates. Making acute hospital services the centerpiece of publicly insured medical care overemphasizes the value of saving and extending lives and sends a signal that the ends realized by other medical acts are merely secondary.[55] The outcome of this line of thinking is that lives should be saved at *all* cost and *regardless* of patients' underlying quality of life. Thus the virtues associated with saving lives become vices when they are allowed to assume an exaggerated importance. Better incorporation of long-term caregiving into the framework of public insurance would demonstrate the importance of neglected values and help to balance the excesses that a more one-sided financing system permits. Since the main aim of caregiving is to enhance individuals' quality of life, financially reimbursing caregiving is one way to infuse this value into health care practice.

A second argument against making individuals and families bear the brunt of financial responsibility for long-term care is that this conflicts with the value of adult independence, which holds that adults are legally, financially, and socially independent unless voluntarily joined together by marriage or responsibility for minor children.[56] Family financial responsibility for the elderly potentially conflicts with this norm by forcing some family members (e.g., adult offspring) to sacrifice on the basis of family relationships that they did not choose to form.

Third, the financial and other costs of caring for elderly individuals should not be assigned primarily to individuals and families because these costs are not spread evenly within the family. Three out of four unpaid caregivers to the elderly are women, usually wives, daughters, and daughters-in-law. Undertaking caregiving activities bears directly on women's lower wages, lower pension earnings, and lower social security benefits. As a result, women who care suffer tremendous financial losses, and nearly one out of three caregivers to the elderly is poor.[57] Divorced, widowed, and separated women are especially vulnerable because they cannot rely on a male wage-earning head of household to share his higher earnings and benefits. Hence, continuing to make families the primary locus of responsibility perpetuates injustices within the family and prevents women from having greater financial and other opportunities.[58] Without dramatic social changes, such as mandating paid employment leave policies, overhauling public and private pension structures, and transforming sexual stereotypes about caregiving, family injustices will persist.

Finally, if society paid for a larger portion of home- and community-based long-term care, this would express societal regard for caregiving. Whereas standing aloof from the financial plight of family caregivers devalues caregiving activity, financially supporting family caregivers renders caregiving less burdensome and more highly esteemed by the society. Furthermore, the love and support family caregivers invest is unlikely to be equaled, even by high quality institutionally based caregivers. Informal caregiving therefore represents a valuable resource that society should protect and strengthen.

Private Financing

To see how we might incorporate these concerns in the financing of long-term care, it is useful to review the major financing alternatives. In 1982 approximately 90 percent of aged persons living in the community with a chronic disability depended on family or friends to remain at home, and 78 percent of this group reported no other caregivers.[59] The labor of informal and unpaid caregivers saves money for public insurers, so government has little incentive to alter the status quo by instituting public policies that provide financial help to families. For example, there is no empirical data to indicate that public policies would increase family caregiving significantly by making families more likely to keep an aging relative at home.[60] Thus it could be argued, from an economic perspective, that investing in informal caregiving is inefficient because it would entail paying a substantial amount for services already supplied at no public cost.

The chief means of financing long-term care in the private sector are paying for long-term care with personal income or using personal resources to purchase private insurance. Self-pay might initially appear to be an attractive option, since on average the real wealth of persons over sixty-five is increasing. However, the incomes and assets of the younger elderly will increase much faster than those of the very old. Moreover, the average nursing home costs of $20,000 to $40,000 per year would bankrupt the majority of Americans within three years.[61] For at least half of the population age sixty-five and over, even if they devoted all of their income to long-term care costs it would cover only about three months of nursing home care for a nonmarried person or nine months of care for a married couple member before impoverishment.[62] Thus if we realistically expect the elderly to pay out of pocket for long-term care, it will be necessary to augment their financial resources, for example, by expanding private pensions, developing a tax-exempt savings program dedicated to long-term care, or making available reverse mortgages to cover long-term care expenses.[63]

Private insurance is an alternative private sector mechanism for funding long-term care. This approach pools the financial resources of many individuals so that the cost of paying for those with long-term care expenses are spread throughout the entire group. Recently, private insurers have become more active in the long-term care market. In 1988 more than 577,000 long-term care policies were bought, bringing the number of these policies to more than one million, compared to only 120,000 policies just five years earlier.[64] Yet despite the recent increase in private insurance for long-term care, long-term care policies remain a tiny portion (less than 1 percent) of the total private health insurance market.[65]

For the foreseeable future there are several reasons for doubting that private insurance can serve as the primary source of financing for long-term care without sacrificing wide access and comprehensive coverage. One problem is adverse selection: the risk of needing long-term care is highly concentrated in a certain subgroup of the elderly that can be readily identified on the basis of age, sex, and functional disability. It is unlikely that those with lesser risk would be willing to subsidize the premiums of others. Without such subsidies, insurers are likely either to exclude persons who have preexisting disabilities or are at risk of developing them, or to charge high premiums beyond the reach of most Americans. At current rates, at most 40 percent and perhaps as few as 6 percent of Americans can afford private long-term care insurance.[66]

A second difficulty with private long-term care insurance is that the package of benefits included in most policies is limited. They are predominantly nursing home or institutional benefits and do not cover community- and home-based care. Where home care is included it is usually offered only in conjunction with more expensive nursing home benefits.[67]

In addition to these points, the arguments presented earlier indicate that bolstering *public* support for family caregiving is a more ethical way of sharing responsibility. The impending crisis in long-term care will enlarge the burden on families, making the need for public support more urgent.

Public Financing

The above discussion makes evident that if society aspires to provide widespread access to comprehensive long-term care and to share fairly the cost of providing these benefits, the public sector will need to play a larger role. In the absence of national health insurance to cover the basic

Nancy S. Jecker

health care needs of all Americans, public policy for long-term care will not be part of an integrated plan in which the value of alternative forms of health care are balanced against each other. Without such a system in place the main alternatives for public financing are expanding current government programs. One strategy consists of covering only those portions of the disabled population unable to obtain private coverage or pay out of pocket. An example of such an approach is expanding Medicaid to cover the entire poor population and to include a more comprehensive package of long-term care benefits. This could be done in conjunction with efforts to promote private long-term care insurance for non-poor citizens. A second strategy is a more far-reaching social program involving the provision of public insurance for long-term care to all older Americans. This might be accomplished through expanding Medicare so that all people over age sixty-five are eligible for long-term care.

In addition to or in place of these alternatives, public financing might be directly targeted to voluntarily initiated family caregiving. One such approach is tax incentives, which would offer economic help without involving government in the actual delivery of care. For example, a tax credit might be introduced that expands the credit for child and dependent care in federal tax law. Such a strategy would require that taxpayers incur employment-related expenses in caring for disabled family members. It would support caregiving expenses irrespective of a family's income, but would place a burden on low-income families by requiring them to incur expenses before receiving credit. An alternative to tax incentives is a direct cash payment to families. At least thirteen states have implemented programs that make direct payments to family caregivers.[68] Funding for them comes from Medicaid and social services block grant monies, as well as state-only funds.

Choosing among feasible strategies for financing long-term care will not be easy. An equitable policy requires that government bear substantially greater financial responsibility for long-term care, support and facilitate family caregiving, and ensure broad access and comprehensive coverage.

Conclusion

I have argued that our society does not devote sufficient resources to long-term care for the chronically disabled elderly. At the same time, we apportion a large share of resources to save and prolong lives. A more equitable means of distributing society's resources must correct this imbalance and place the good of improving life's quality alongside the value of extending life. Rather than separating caregiving activities from formal distributive programs, such activities should be better integrated into insurance frameworks. Rather than leaving the costs of long-term care to be borne by individuals and families, the public should play a more active and supportive role.

In closing, it is important to note and underscore that a just system for *financing* long-term care is only a first step toward a more comprehensive long-term care plan. More equitable financing of long-term care does not yet begin to address further questions about the proper structuring and delivery of these services. Merely gaining access to long-term care hardly guarantees that the self-respect and dignity of individuals will be furthered. To the contrary, some studies show that the very act of allowing someone else to do something for one can erode self-respect and self-determination by leading people to infer that they are more helpless than they in fact are.[69] In one study of institutionalized elderly people, "helping" interventions actually reduced subjects' ability to perform tasks independently, increased their perception of task difficulty, and reduced their confidence about independently performing tasks.[70] This suggests that long-term care can induce greater dependency and thwart the very values it is designed to protect.

If even good-intentioned caregivers' efforts can introduce iatrogenic disabilities, then putting a just system of long-term care in place will require considerable attention to the delivery, as well as the financing, of long-term care services. Although the benefits of an improved system will be felt most directly by disabled persons, we all share a common stake in creating and supporting a more just and compassionate community. The ephemerality of youthful independence and vigor make it prudent, as well as right and compassionate, to improve the financing and delivery of long-term care. There is no good reason to postpone this effort, and no means of justifying our continued neglect of disabled elderly people.

Notes

This essay draws on a keynote address that I delivered for the 1992 Conference on Cardiovascular Health and Disease in Women, National Institutes of Health, National Heart, Lung and Blood Institute, Bethesda, Maryland.

Earlier versions were presented to the University of Toronto Centre for Bioethics in February 1992 and to the NEH Conference on "Rationing Health Care: Ethics and Aging" in March 1992. I am grateful to various individuals who provided helpful feedback on this essay, especially Professor Carroll Estes, Albert Jonsen, and Eric Meslin.

1. Daniel Callahan, *Setting Limits: Medical Goals in an Aging Society* (New York: Simon and Schuster, 1987); Timothy M. Smeeding, ed., *Should Medical Care Be Rationed by Age?* (Towtowa, N.J.: Rowman and Littlefield, 1987), xi–xv; Samuel Preston, "Children and the Elderly in the U.S.," *Scientific American* 251 (1984): 44–49; Norman Daniels, *Am I My Parents' Keeper? An Essay on Justice between the Young and the Old* (New York: Oxford University Press, 1988); Paul Menzel, *Medical Costs, Moral Choices: A Philosophy of Health Care Economics in America* (New Haven: Yale University Press, 1983); Robert H. Binstock and Steven G. Post, eds., *Too Old for Health Care? Controversies in Medicine, Law, Economics, and Ethics* (Baltimore: Johns Hopkins University Press, 1991); Paul Homer and Martha Holstein, eds., *A Good Old Age?* (New York: Simon and Schuster, 1991); Nancy S. Jecker and R. A. Pearlman, "Ethical Constraints on Rationing Medical Care by Age," *Journal of the American Geriatrics Society* 37 (1989): 1067–75; Nancy S. Jecker, "Disenfranchising the Elderly from Life-Extending Medical Care," *Public Affairs Quarterly* 2 (1988): 51–68; Norman G. Levinsky, "Age as a Criterion for Rationing Health Care," *New England Journal of Medicine* 322 (1990): 1813–16; Mark Siegler, "Should Age Be a Criterion for Rationing Health Care?" *Hastings Center Report* 14 (1984): 24–27.

2. Edward L. Schneider and Jack M. Guralnik, "The Aging of America: Impact on Health Care Costs," *Journal of the American Medical Association* 263 (1990): 2335–40.

3. Nancy S. Jecker, "Age-Based Rationing and Women," *Journal of the American Medical Association* 266 (1991): 3012–15.

4. Amy M. Haddad and Marshall B. Kapp, "Economics and Ethics," in Amy M. Haddad and Marshall B. Kapp, eds., *Ethical and Legal Issues in Home Health Care* (Norwalk, Conn.: Appleton and Lange, 1991), 101–20.

5. President's Commission for the Study of Ethical Problems in Medicine and Biomedical and Behavioral Research, *Securing Access to Health Care*, vol. 1 (Washington, D.C.: Government Printing Office, 1983).

6. Diane Rowland and Barbara Lyons, "The Elderly Population in Need of Home Care," in Diane Rowland and Barbara Lyons, eds., *Financing Home Care* (Baltimore: Johns Hopkins University Press, 1991), 3–26.

7. Institute of Medicine, *Toward a National Strategy for Long-Term Care of*

the Elderly: A Study Plan for Evaluation of New Polity Options for the Future (Washington, D.C.: National Academy of Sciences, 1986).

8. Older Women's League, "The Picture of Health in Mid-life and Older Women," *Women and Health* 14 (1988): 53–73.

9. Peter W. Shaughnessy and Andrew M. Kramer, "The Increased Needs of Patients in Nursing Homes and Patients Receiving Home Health Care," *New England Journal of Medicine* 322 (1990): 21–27.

10. Eileen Chichin, "Community Care for the Frail Elderly: The Case of Non-Professional Home Care Workers," *Women and Health* 14 (1988): 93–104. The remaining funding sources include social service block grants, Older American's Act grants, and states. The Veteran's Administration also finances home care on a limited basis following acute illness.

11. Judith Feder, "Paying for Home Care: The Limits of Current Programs," in Rowland and Lyons, eds., *Financing Home Care,* 27–50.

12. Ernest M. Gruenberg, "The Failures of Success," *Milbank Memorial Fund Quarterly: Health and Society* 55 (1977): 3–24.

13. Council on Scientific Affairs, American Medical Association, "AMA White Paper on Elderly Health," *Archives of Internal Medicine* 150 (1990): 2459–72.

14. Terry Todd Wetle, "Ethical Aspects of Decision Making for and with the Elderly," in Marshall B. Kapp, Harvey E. Pies, A. Edward Doudera, eds., *Legal and Ethical Aspects of Health Care for the Elderly* (Ann Arbor: Health Administration Press, 1985), 258–68.

15. Lois M. Verbrugge, "An Epidemiological Profile of Older Women," in Marie R. Haug, Amassa B. Ford, and Marian Shaefor, eds., *The Physical and Mental Health of Aged Women* (New York: Springer, 1985), 41–64.

16. Older Women's League, "Picture of Health."

17. Ibid.

18. Verbrugge, "Epidemiological Profile."

19. Ibid.

20. Ibid.

21. Ibid.

22. Shoshanna Sofaer and Emily Abel, "Older Women's Health and Financial Vulnerability," *Women and Health* 16:3–4 (1990): 47–67.

23. Older Women's League, "Picture of Health."

24. Meredith Minkler and R. Stone, "The Feminization of Poverty and Older Women," *The Gerontologist* 25 (1985): 351–57.

25. Ethel D. Kahn, "The Women's Movement and Older Women's Health," *Women and Health* 9 (1984): 87–100.

26. Sofaer and Abel, "Older Women's Health."

27. L. Gregory Pawlson, "Financing Long-Term Care: The Growing Dilemma," *Journal of the American Geriatrics Society* 37 (1989): 631–38.

28. Minkler and Stone, "Feminization of Poverty."

29. Christine K. Cassel and Bernice L. Neugarten, "A Forecast of Women's Health and Longevity: Implications for an Aging America," *Western Journal of Medicine* 149 (1988): 712–17.

30. Institute of Medicine, *Toward a National Strategy for Long-Term Care of the Elderly: A Study Plan for Evaluation of New Polity Options for the Future* (Washington, D.C.: National Academy of Sciences, 1986).

31. These figures are reported in M. Lewis, "Health Needs of Women as They Age," *Women and Health* 10 (1985): 1–16. All figures assume that immigration, emigration, birth, and mortality rates remain relatively predictable.

32. Claudia Mills, "The Graying of America," *Report from the Institute for Philosophy and Public Policy* 8 (1988): 1–5.

33. U.S. Bureau of the Census, Office of the Actuary, *The Centenarians* (Washington, D.C.: Government Printing Office, 1988).

34. Dennis F. Johnson and Sally L. Hoover, "Social Indicators of Aging," in Matilda White Riley, Ronald P. Ables, and Michael S. Teitelbaum, eds., *Aging from Birth to Death*, vol. 2: *Socioeconomic Perspectives* (Boulder: Westview, 1982).

35. Mills, "Graying of America."

36. Council on Scientific Affairs, "AMA White Paper."

37. Sofaer and Abel, "Older Women's Health."

38. James F. Fries, "The Compression of Morbidity," *Milbank Memorial Fund Quarterly: Health and Society* 61 (1983): 397–419.

39. Preston, "Children and the Elderly."

40. Older Women's League, *Failing America's Caregivers: A Status Report on Women Who Care* (Washington, D.C.: Older Women's League, 1989), 1–12.

41. Ibid.

42. Arthur Caplan, "The Morality of the Mundane: Ethical Issues Arising in the Daily Lives of Nursing Home Residents," in R. A. Kane and A. L. Caplan, eds., *Everyday Ethics: Resolving Dilemmas in Nursing Home Life* (New York: Springer, 1990), 21–36.

43. John Rawls, *A Theory of Justice* (Cambridge: Harvard University Press, 1971), 440.

44. Thomas E. Hill, *Autonomy and Self-Respect* (New York: Cambridge University Press, 1991).

45. Amy Gutmann, "For and against Equal Access to Health Care," in Pres-

ident's Commission for the Study of Biomedical and Behavioral Research, *Securing Access to Health Care,* vol. 2 (Washington, D.C.: Government Printing Office, 1983), 51–66.

46. Judith N. Shklar, *The Faces of Injustice* (New Haven: Yale University Press, 1990), 38.

47. Aristotle, *Nicomachean Ethics,* in Richard McKeon, ed., *The Basic Works of Aristotle* (New York: Random House, 1941), 1001.

48. Albert Jonsen, "Resentment and the Rights of the Elderly," in Nancy S. Jecker, ed., *Aging and Ethics* (Clifton, N.J.: Humana Press, 1991), 341–52.

49. James S. Benson and Kevin J. Kennelly, "Learned Helplessness: The Result of Uncontrollable Reinforcements or Uncontrollable Aversive Stimuli?" *Journal of Personality and Society Psychology* 34 (1976): 138–45; S. F. Maier and M. E. P. Seligman, "Learned Helplessness: Theory and Evidence," *Journal of Experimental Psychology: General* 103 (1976): 3–46.

50. As Eric Meslin, and several other Canadians who heard this essay, pointed out to me, Canada and many other industrialized countries have long recognized long-term care as a requirement of justice. For example, Canada has had programs that provide universal entitlement to nursing home care in place since the 1970s, and all but the poorest of its provinces provide financial coverage for necessary care in a nursing home regardless of a person's income or assets. For more on this point, see Rosalie Kane and Robert Kane, "Home- and Community-Based Care in Canada," in Rowland and Lyons, eds., *Financing Home Care,* 199–228.

51. Aristotle, *Nicomachean Ethics,* 1003.

52. Rawls, *Theory of Justice,* 440; Sharon Bishop Hill, "Self-Determination and Autonomy," in Richard A. Wasserstrom, ed., *Today's Moral Problems* (New York: Macmillan, 1979), 118–33.

53. See Pawlson, "Financing Long-Term Care."

54. Institute of Medicine, *Toward a National Strategy.*

55. Christine K. Cassel and Bernice L. Neugarten, "The Goals of Medicine in an Aging Society," in Binstock and Post, eds., *Too Old for Health Care?* 75–91.

56. Alice M. Rivlin and Joshua M. Wiener, *Caring for the Disabled Elderly: Who Will Pay?* (Washington, D.C.: Brookings Institution, 1988).

57. Older Women's League, *Failing America's Caregivers.*

58. Nancy S. Jecker, "What Do Husbands and Wives Owe Each Other in Old Age?" in Lawrence B. McCullough and Nancy L. Wilson, eds., *Long-Term Care Decisions* (Baltimore: Johns Hopkins University Press, 1995), 155–80.

59. Jonsen, "Resentment and the Rights of the Elderly."

60. Ibid.

61. Charlene Harrington, Christine Cassel, Carroll Estes, et al., "A National Long-Term Care Program for the United States," *Journal of the American Medical Association* 266 (1991): 3023–29.

62. Institute of Medicine, *Toward a National Strategy.*

63. Stanley S. Wallack, "Alternative Methods of Financing Long-Term Care," in Kapp et al., eds., *Legal and Ethical Aspects of Health Care,* 73–82.

64. Milt Freudenheim, "Long-Term Care Policies Improve," *New York Times,* Feb. 7, 1989, C-28.

65. Charlene Harrington and Steffie Woolhandler, "Working Group on Long-Term Care Program Design—Physicians for a National Health Program: A National Long-Term Care Program for the United States," *Journal of the American Medical Association* 266 (1991): 3023–29.

66. Aristotle, *Nicomachean Ethics,* 1001.

67. Diane Rowland and Barbara Lyons, "A Proposal to Expand Home Care Benefits," in Rowland and Lyons, eds., *Financing Home Care,* 229–47.

68. Jonsen, "Resentment and the Rights of the Elderly."

69. Ellen J. Langer, *The Psychology of Control* (Beverly Hills: Sage, 1983), 101–16; Judith Rodin, "Control by Any Other Name," in Judith Rodin, Carmi Schooler, K. Warner Schaie, eds., *Self-Directedness: Cause and Effects throughout the Life Course* (Hillsdale, N.J.: Lawrence Erlbaum Associates, 1990), 1–18.

70. Langer, *Psychology of Control,* 271–78.

Part 3

Reflections

5

Bioethics in a Disposable Society
Health Care and the Intergenerational Stake

Carroll L. Estes, Susan E. Kelly, and Elizabeth A. Binney

Social Science and Bioethics: Reexamining Assumptions

Social science contributions to bioethical analysis can occur in a variety
of ways, generally falling under one of two overarching approaches. Social scientists can bring into central focus those contextual variables that
form the "real world" of health care policy and delivery. They can also
contribute a framework or vision that problematizes the subject matter
of bioethical analysis, yielding alternative perspectives in the activity of
asking, and answering, normative questions.

This essay is addressed to the latter goal. We raise the question of probable or potential social and policy influences flowing from the applied
philosophical debate concerned with the moral justification of age-based
rationing of health care. We suggest a basis for this impact through the
sociological perspective of social construction in the context of power,
policy, and discourse. This approach attends to the bioethical age-rationing debate as an ineluctably meaningful social form, itself implicated in
the processes of assigning meaning to the complex social reality of health
care. We suggest that development of a discourse of moral justification
for a policy option embedded within a particular construction of reality,
by a field that from its inception has been no stranger to policy, may enhance the legitimacy of that policy approach.

The potential legitimating role of applied philosophy implies that critical attention to the underlying assumptions of a debate should precede
the development of moral theory. We will examine the assumptions of
crisis and scarcity in health care and their relationship to elderly consumers. We conclude that bioethics, at its boundaries with public policy, may

benefit from the incorporation of critical contextual analysis of dominant assumptions that can set the agenda of ethical argument and affect even the selection of topics and problems to be discussed.[1]

Several features of bioethical discourse on age rationing may shape its potential for social influence. These include a tendency toward abstraction from empirical social structures, interests, and processes; a focus on individuals relatively unconstrained by the effects of social structure in models of decision making; and the obscuring of ideology as a consequence of the rational deductive methodology for developing normative and moral systems.

We juxtapose a conflict model of policy formation to the individual-centered model that places agency with reasoned decision makers in an idealized, abstracted context of information and choice. We seek to redirect analytical attention to the structural forces that create the contexts constraining individual decision making, and that drive inequalities and irrationalities in health care production and delivery. We postulate that the definitions of social reality that underlie arguments for age rationing reflect the interests and ideologies of their producers.

Thus we are "critical" of the claims of resource scarcity that support a causal link between demand and consumption of health care by the elderly and escalating national health care costs. That scarcity itself has not been put through the requirements of rigorous definition. Which resources are scarce, and which in over-supply? Do we know enough about the causes of scarcity to conclude that they would be substantially alleviated by restricting access to health care by age? Or is scarcity caused by deeper irrationalities in our current system that would continue to drive costs up and expand use?

The rising costs of health care over the past two decades have provided the primary impetus to age-rationing debates. Cost increases, however, are attributable to a wide range of causal factors. Approximately 55 percent of the increase, for instance, can be attributed to population growth and general inflation.[2] Medical care price inflation accounted for 17 percent, and the volume and intensity of services for approximately 28 percent of the increase. Growth in these components has been affected by factors including: increased patient complexity; a tendency in the delivery system toward specialization rather than primary care; concentration of physicians and hospitals in certain urban areas, leading to excess capacity and lower productivity while other areas are underserved;

unnecessary and inappropriate care, which some estimate may be as high as 25 percent of health care services; the practice of defensive medicine to avoid the threat of malpractice suits; and excessive administrative costs.[3]

Although we would like to see increased reflexivity about the policy role of bioethics, we recognize all too well how difficult it is to achieve in any disciplinary endeavor. Yet as scholars and writers analyzing a controversy, we are nourishing it: we are performing a consequential act.[4]

Health Care versus Medical Care: Political Economy and Generational Equity

Three basic aspects of the perspective we are suggesting should be stated from the outset. First, in discussions of rationing and resource allocation, use of the term "health care" inaccurately frames the debate. The term "health care" is often used when what is discussed is more accurately "medical care"—the acute care, high technology, and medical services and procedures associated with the practice of modern medicine. This narrow meaning ignores the vast majority of the care and resources that the elderly (and other vulnerable population groups such as children) most need—public health measures including housing and nutrition, preventive care, chronic care, long-term care, and health promotion services—and that are beyond the scope of much of what is termed "health care" in our society. Thus insofar as the debate about "health care" rationing is only about "medical care," many, if not most, of the health needs of the elderly are ignored. This semantic difference can be significant when the costs associated with medical and health care are examined. The U.S. Congress Office of Technology Assessment, for instance, reported in 1987 that only a small proportion of nursing home patients, who account for roughly 21 percent of elderly health care expenditures, are treated with life-sustaining technologies (mechanical ventilation, resuscitation, and nutritional support through tube or intravenous feeding). Nonhospital and nonphysician health services—such items as prescription drugs, dental care, and home health care—and physician fees for out- and in-patient services comprise 38 percent; and payments to hospitals comprise the remaining 41 percent.[5] In a study of medical care in the last twelve months of life, Scitovsky found that hospital costs for the elderly were less than half of those for younger age groups in the study.[6] While nursing home and home health care expenditures were higher in the oldest group (eighty and over), these increases were offset by declines in hospital and physician costs in the last year of life. These are among data[7] supporting the alternative interpretation that the elderly are not disproportionate users of high technology, high cost aggressive "health care" measures.

Second, the present social, cultural, political, and economic environment represents a dynamic and determining set of influences not only in the production of social issues and social policy, but also in the disciplinary discourse of bioethics. The political economy theoretical lens orients analysis toward gender, race/ethnicity, and class as major, determining (rather than contextual) variables. Encompassing social, cultural, and political forces must be treated as both "real" and significant influences in the bioethics debate. "Society," "culture," and "environment" are not mere passive background or contextual variables, but are considered essential and integral to any analysis of the health care rationing debate concerning the aging.

Third, bioethics discourse on aging and medical care is imbued with questions of generational equity, posed in terms of moral rights and responsibilities regarding societal resources.[8] We use the term "intergenerational stake" to challenge the rhetoric of intergenerational trade-offs. Images and metaphors of "greedy geezers" mortgaging the future of the young are powerful symbolic weapons that may be used to further political and economic ends. The deployment of such symbols can shape public policy and the allocation of resources that create and maintain various strata within society.

The view of the aged as a "disposable" burden to society diverts attention from the externally determined factors that lead to financial dependence of the elderly. These include their high and growing out-of-pocket health and medical care costs, the inadequacy of Medicare, the insistence of policy makers that elders rely on an aggressively profit-oriented private insurance market to provide Medigap insurance, and declining employment opportunities even until age sixty-five.[9] Further social causes of old age dependency encompass social policies and practices that promote age discrimination and (until recently) mandatory retirement; lower incomes of retired persons that decline with age; the treatment of functional disability and chronic illness with acute medical care rather than rehabilitative and personal support; social isolation; the low self-esteem resulting from the stigmatized status of older persons; and the asymmetrical power relations between older persons and professional caregivers.[10] Further, this view ignores the differential life course consequences of such social structural factors as class for health. A life of poverty is highly correlated with ill health and chronic illness (and health care requirements) in later years. Individual and group differences in lifetime opportunities (a structural problem) translate into differences in vulnerability and dependency throughout the life course.

Setting the Agenda: Crisis Construction and the Emergence of Age-Rationing Literature

The Social Construction of Crisis in Health and Aging

The social construction of crises and the designation of such issues as aging and health care as fundamentally threatening national problems illustrate what Berger and Luckmann have called the "social construction of reality."[11] A perceived reality becomes solidified, and consequential, when people act as if it were real. Policy action and social consequences flow from such definitions and perceptions, although they may only represent partial "realities." The social construction of reality about old age and health has provided a legitimating rationale that serves as a basis for public policy within these areas.

Three major constructions underlie the political economy of health and aging in our society. Aging tends to be characterized as a process of biological and physiological decline; some elderly are seen as "deserving" while others are not; and old age and old people are seen as a social problem. Further, the old age problem is defined as being one of crisis proportions.[12] It is in this context that care for the elderly is seen to be a major contributing factor to the health care crisis and the one for which rationing solutions are most readily sought.

Social, economic, and political stakes are invested in the definition and perception of social problems and whether or not they are defined as crises.[13] While organized interests play a complex role in crisis construction, a variety of social institutions may function to legitimate that construction.[14] These institutions may include not only the major structural forces of the economy, religion, and government but also those that produce undergirding systems of thought or rationale. As the field assumes a more prominent role in health policy debate, bioethics may hold the potential for having this effect; in treating a crisis construction, or a causal imputation, as real, by developing moral theory directed toward solutions of the crisis or dilemma, bioethics may participate in solidification of that reality construction.

We have been criticized in this position for both imputing that bioethicists are merely the producers of rhetoric and for suggesting that social problems such as the confluence of an aging society and health care crisis would cease to exist with a change of perception. In answer to the first point, our suggestion that a gulf exists between abstract solutions and the practical existence of a problem need not be coincident with the claim that the theory lacks substance. The development of moral theory may not be rooted in praxis, but it is not beyond the realm of intended or unintended effects. Applied ethics may be abstracted from context yet directed toward practice. The rules and principles from which moral systems are built determine how moral problems are formulated because they provide the criteria for ascertaining what features of the world are morally relevant.[15] It is this determination of morally relevant features from among the complex network of associations and causalities involved in health policy that may render bioethical theory development justifying a particular policy construction a compelling form of legitimation.[16] Social constructionism holds that social forms are ineluctably meaningful, and the process of assigning meaning is a practical and integral element of the form's social reality. With political economy, the perspective underscores the dialectical relationship between ideas and values that are identified and legitimated in the formulation of public policy as dominant, as "right" and consensually held, and public acceptance of those values. This process is of special interest in the examination of an enterprise such as bioethics, where the intellectual community is explicitly involved in value construction and clarification in a public policy context. We are suggesting that, rather than the lack of direct influence on policy lamented by some in the bioethics community,[17] bioethical discourse may play an unintended role by legitimating dominant, and unexamined, assumptions about sociopolitical reality.

Regarding the second point, by suggesting deeper examination of the assumptions driving claims for the necessity of rationing medical care by age, rather than refinement of arguments about age rationing, we are suggesting that other mechanisms for controlling the rise in health care costs be addressed seriously before age rationing is seen as necessary or acceptable. Determination of these mechanisms should begin by examining the structural interests supported by the production of health care needs and services and focusing on the resolution of irrationalities in the market system for services.

The Emergence of Age-Rationing Literature

Following the passage of Medicare and Medicaid in 1965, health care costs rose dramatically at two to four times the inflation rate. Although the 1960s were devoted to struggles about rights and equality of access, this brief progressive interlude abruptly ended with the oil shocks of the 1970s and the dawning of the United States' economic decline in the world order. Economic issues eclipsed the nation's concern with health care access. In its place, the 1970s was the period in which comprehensive health care, systems development, and the rationalization of health planning were to "solve" the problem of rising costs.[18] At the same time, the search for scapegoats was beginning, with entitlement programs such as Medicare as prime candidates. In 1979 Joseph Califano, then Secretary of the Department of Health, Education, and Welfare, coined the phrase, the "graying of the budget," following Samuelson's volatile and important treatise in the *National Journal* on "Busting the U.S. Budget: The Costs of an Aging America."[19] The predictable failure of voluntary hospital cost containment during the Carter presidency set the stage for the 1980s, in which the fixation with controlling health costs would be joined with the rhetoric of individual responsibility, privatization, competition, and deregulation. Reagan's victory was not just at the polls, it was in installing and utilizing the theme of crisis as a central motif of his presidency.[20] With the crisis theme came the ideology of austerity and the politics of unequal sacrifice. In health care the crisis construction and its political uses were focused on cost containment. Describing the early Reagan years, Estes observes that

> Perhaps the most serious potential threat to the survival of a viable public policy for the elderly is the construction of reality that links the perception of fiscal crisis with an aging society. This perception is promoted by . . . popular periodicals . . . [that portray] the "graying" federal budget as a major source of the nation's economic troubles. Of great concern to the aging will be the outcome of power struggles among contending views concerning the needs of the aged, their rights, and their social responsibilities.[21]

It should come as no surprise, then, that when Allen Greenspan told the Health Insurance Association of America in 1983 that 28 percent of

Medicare dollars were being spent annually on about 6 percent of Medicare-eligible individuals who die within the year, the concept of rationing health care services to the elderly was on its way to legitimacy.

The 1980s were also a period during which inequities in Medicare benefits for the low-income and minority elderly were exacerbated, particularly for the near-poor elderly, by changes in health policy justified by rising health care costs and budget cuts. Budget cuts of nearly $18 billion by the end of 1985 increased the proportion of costs paid by Medicare recipients, with economic hardship falling to those least able to bear it. In the context of a $4,226 median income for the elderly in 1980, in 1981 health care costs exceeded $1,100 in per capital out-of-pocket costs, and continued to rise.[22] Both deductibles and co-payments increased dramatically: a 27 percent increase in the Part A deductible between 1981 and 1982 and a 25 percent increase in the Part B deductible during the same period. Increased cost sharing was instituted in a number of areas under Medicare, expanding class, race, and gender based inequities. These consequences for the elderly have been attributed to the U.S. commitment, reflected in public policy, to the market ideology, to individualism, and to competition.[23]

The 1980s were also a period of change for bioethics. A major issue raised internally by bioethicists in the 1980s was how to modulate the principle of autonomy with other significant social values—societal questions of community and interdependence.[24] In June 1984, the Hastings Center organized a symposium on "Autonomy, Paternalism, and Community" in honor of its fifteenth anniversary.[25] The symposium presented a forum for discussions about a new dominant theme in bioethics, the just distribution of resources.[26] The move into the area of large-scale health care delivery and policy issues gained notoriety beyond the immediate discipline with the age-rationing proposal put forward by Daniel Callahan in Setting Limits: Medical Goals in an Aging Society (1987). His proposal spawned an expansive debate within the field of bioethics over age-based health care rationing schemes, and just intergenerational distributions of societal resources in general.

Callahan's original proposal was an expression of his interest in correcting what some saw as the overemphasis of bioethics on individualism and an inability to express a "morality in the company of others, community as an ideal, and interdependence as a perceived reality."[27] He suggested a societal reorientation in the meaning of aging and the personal rewards appropriate to the later phase of life. This proposed shift in values was welded to his concerns about exploding medical care costs and crises of resource allocation. His suggested linking of these issues, a search for meaning based on community rather than the individual and the economically rationalized search for modes of restricting consumption of medical care, helped shape a moral discourse coincident with the political framework of the 1980s. That is, as health policy discussion centered ever more firmly on the elderly in terms of cost-containment and entitlement reduction, a bioethics overshadowed by "autonomy's temporary triumph"[28] was in danger of becoming increasingly marginal. What emerged was a multifaceted dialogue within bioethics concerning normative claims and obligations specific to age, and moral justification for cost-containment solutions based on claims of age-specific consumption of medical resources. The bioethics dialogue developed as the moral characterization of what we have defined as a political, rather than merely empirical, discourse.

Rationality and Moral Problem Solving

While the content of bioethics may have shifted over the past decade away from essential individualism, the method employed by bioethicists such as Menzel and Daniels (for example, in this volume) in the development of arguments about age and resources has remained true to analytic philosophy.[29] This methodology has been variously characterized: as rational abstraction,[30] leading to the isolation of issues from their concrete human reality; and as "doing morality."[31]

Hoffmaster finds fault with three features of the deductive model dominating the academic literature of applied ethics: imperviousness to the contexts in which moral problems arise, a static conception of moral problem solving, and reliance on a formal notion of rationality, such that rationality engenders normativity. Relating his first point to the present subject—bioethical arguments concerning rationing medical resources by age—we suggest that the contexts in which moral problems arise include the macro-ideological contexts of political discourse. Critical theory seeks to identify the interests that benefit from interpretations of reality, particularly interpretations that seek to "blame" vulnerable groups for systemic problems, or that appeal inconsistently to limits (e.g., political uses of crisis).

The context within which moral problems addressed by applied ethics are defined is re-constructed in order to isolate relevant variables: values, conflicts, norms. It is the construction of the problem that makes the solution so compelling. For example, Menzel's abstracted, idealized insurance paradigm, while not conforming to the empirical constraints experienced by decision-making consumers, provides the appropriate structure for the logistical deductivism of his argument.

The technique that leads from rationality to morality is expressed by Hoffmaster in the following passage:

> Philosophers are not satisfied with answers to the question, "But why *ought* I to do that?" that appeal to considerations such as the prospect of a social sanction being imposed, de facto beliefs of the community about what is good or right, or the wishes of someone in a position of power, because these are not legitimate *moral* answers. Such concerns may, in fact, motivate people to do what they ought to do; nevertheless, they are spurious sources of normativity. Philosophers are happier with an answer that attempts to provide a rational ground or warrant for moral norms because if these norms express what rationality prescribes, and if human beings are rational creatures, then it follows that human beings *ought* to obey them. The rationality involved in the construction of a consistent, coherent system of valid moral norms is taken to engender normativity.[32]

Further, rational agents are expected to act to maximize their expected subjective utility. Rationality in this sense also leads to an affinity with the decision-making processes assumed by economists: the rational, informed person will enter the marketplace seeking to maximize transactional gains and minimize losses. These properties are troubling when considering concepts such as Menzel's hypothetical prudent consent: he seems to be arguing that within certain conditions we can presume the person for whom we are hypothesizing decision-making would have acted within our own normative constraints of rationality. The assumption of rationality is itself class-based, as it has been criticized for being gender based;[33] applying prudence implies both forms of rationality and real choices that are available differentially within the social order.

Health Care Rationing: Crisis and Contradiction

At 14 percent ($817 billion) of the gross national product in 1992 with projections of growth to $1.472 trillion by 1997,[34] medical expenditures contribute to one of the few "healthy" areas of our current economy in terms of both investment capital return and employment. The passage of Medicare and Medicaid in 1965 and its subsequent structural configuration fueled explosive growth in for-profit components and the costs of a gigantic medical-industrial complex.[35]

In 1988, approximately 40 percent of the cost of U.S health care is publicly financed by the state.[36] These expenditures have underwritten a panoply of largely private-sector providers and medical industries, while the public sector has limited its activities in health and social services to those that complement and support the market through the public financing of health insurance.[37] These structural arrangements stimulate market investment opportunities for business in areas that promise the greatest likelihood of profit (e.g., hospital and home health services, pharmaceuticals, medical equipment). State policy also promotes productive opportunities for business through civil law and regulation protecting the market and encouraging the entry of proprietary providers in areas of health care where they previously were barred from receiving reimbursement. In the late 1980s, President Bush's proposed federal tax subsidy for the purchase of private health insurance attempted to combine policies to promote private enterprise with a solution to health access problems.

State actions and policies have thus contributed to: (1) the deepening of divisions in the de facto rationing system of U.S. health care based on ability to pay;[38] and (2) a largely unchecked rise in federal medical care costs. As Estes observes, U.S. health and aging policy exemplifies "the contradictions facing the state as it tries to simultaneously regulate and contain government costs in medical care and to deregulate and promote economic expansion and profit through a robust, privately-run and extremely costly medical-industrial complex."[39] This is the context of the rationing debate of the 1980s and early 1990s, including proposals for the explicit rationing of health care by age.

Changing Foci of Cost Containment

The literature emerging in the wake of Callahan's suggestions, and which is the subject of this essay, has tended to maintain the crux of the economic solution: the individual elderly consumer. This focus may reflect the fact that other mechanisms for containing costs may be more difficult to measure or even to define, where statistics on resource utilization and aggregate costs under Medicare were readily available and visible. Data that appeared to link resource demands by the elderly and the increasing costs of societal aging to the perceived health care crisis were widely quoted.[40] Relevant studies indicated that a large fraction of hospital costs incurred by high-cost Medicare patients are attributable to patients who die during their hospitalization or shortly thereafter.[41] Others showed that a small fraction (6 percent) of Medicare beneficiaries who died accounted for 28 percent of Medicare reimbursements in 1978.[42] In addition, the proportion of the gross national product consumed by health care in 1987 was nearly double what it was in 1965, the year Medicare was enacted.[43]

Directing cost-containment attention to the health services market has been more difficult conceptually and in policy terms, although this trend may be changing. Medical technological innovation and inappropriate or ineffective use of technologies have recently begun to be examined for their contributions to rising health care costs. Addressing the roles of technology production and physician practice patterns is an analytical approach less amenable to rationing solutions concentrating on individual consumer behavior and characteristics. It will be much more difficult, although more steps are being taken in this direction, to be "prudent" in the production and use of expensive medical commodities of unproven value than to develop prudent schemes for the individual use of all existing technologies.

During the mid-1970s, concern for the effects of medical technology on health care costs was high.[44] The National Center for Health Care Technology, no longer in existence, was legislated to address this concern, and the Sun Valley Forum in 1977 produced a seminal review of the issue by Stanley Wallack and Stuart Altman. The 1980s witnessed relatively little attention to the issue, in part because of the difficulties of conceptualizing the problem, and likely in part because consumer-level rationing had been successfully defined as a logical and necessary policy direction. An Institute of Medicine (IOM) meeting in 1992 concluded that the conceptual basis for analyzing the relationship between technology and health care expenditures had not advanced sufficiently to warrant further review. It was concluded by the participants, mostly health economists, that it would be useful to examine the economic reasons why information about the effectiveness of technology was not being generated at an adequate level, as well as to examine the political reaction within the private sector to the creation of such information. More recently, however, a general consensus has emerged that a significant share of annual real health care cost growth is attributable to medical technology.

Joseph Newhouse has attempted to quantify the contributions of possible causes of spending growth, including an aging population, health insurance, physician-induced demand, defensive medicine, administrative costs, and the costs of caring for the terminally ill in the last year of life.[45] He argues that, rather than these factors, it is the residual attributable to the increased capabilities of medicine and the continued progress of science that accounts for much of the increase in health care expenditures.

In addition to their growth, the effectiveness and appropriate use of medical technologies is also difficult to evaluate. Roos and Roos argue that there is little hard evidence available to evaluate the effectiveness of many medical acts and procedures, within or outside of the acute care sector, including the commonplace, the high tech, the expensive, and the new.[46] Without such evidence, opinions within the medical profession vary widely about appropriate treatment and diagnosis, and the use of interventions varies significantly among regions, hospitals, and physicians. Analyses of appropriate use and discretion based on expert opinion have shown high levels of inappropriate and equivocal medical decision making, both when looking at individual procedures and in general reviews of hospital use.[47] Establishing measures of cost-effectiveness, as in terms of cost per quality-adjusted life-year, is made problematic by poor, biased, and incommensurable data. Population-based, nonrandomized data is scarce. Patient preferences for treatment, presumably a significant factor in age-rationing proposals such as Callahan's and in different ways, both Menzel's and Daniel's, appear to follow a pattern of risk aversion. Patients also tend to choose differently than their doctors when given a choice.[48] Both patients and physicians, however, appear to contribute to the trend for low-risk diagnostic procedures, providing better information if not treatment, and driving interest in such technologies as magnetic resonance imaging (MRI), endoscopy, extra consultations, and laboratory testing.

Finally, Blustein and Marmor[49] make a significant point regarding efforts to reduce "waste" by making rules to limit the use of beneficial services (i.e., rationing): the *perception* of benefit determines the *political* cost of rationing. Likewise, the perception of cost is significant to the reception of rationing proposals. These facts underline the potential influence of analyses that assume or generalize about the costs and benefits of allowing access to particular medical technologies by particular individuals.

Thus the 1980s experienced a confluence of factors supporting age-rationing solutions to the perceived health care system crisis: the political construction of aging as a social problem; the emergence and expansion of age-based alternatives in the bioethics literature; and the lack of available mechanisms for quantifying the contribution of medical innovation and ineffective or inappropriate uses of medical technology on health care costs.

Bioethics and Public Policy: A Complex Relationship

An area of tension has been identified between the practice of "applied ethics" as an intellectual activity and the involvement of ethicists in the public policy process.[50] The establishment of the legitimacy of "applied ethics" as an intellectual activity and the appropriate roles, stance, and goals of ethicists in the public policy arena are issues of continuing debate within the field. The literature concerning the relationship of professional philosophy and its practitioners to the processes of public policy formulation evidences growing recognition that the impact of bioethics scholarship on social institutions and policy may be indirect, ancillary to other agendas and processes, and may potentially lead to unforeseen or undesired outcomes.[51] A goal in our present analysis is to encourage the reflexive position in professional bioethics, including consideration of social and political processes to which the field is inevitably joined.

Although debate existed in the early development of modern bioethics (1960s and 1970s) concerning the allocation of health care resources, the issues were focused primarily on emerging technologies and the scarcity of resources such as organs for transplantation.[52] The emergence of age-related rationing in bioethical discourse occurred in conjunction not only with Reagan-era cost containment in social spending, but with perceptions of and legislative actions directed toward fiscal crises in both Social Security and Medicare.[53] New cost-containment initiatives, including implementation of the prospective payment system, threatened both the autonomy and fiscal security of established medical care providers, many of whom relied heavily on government spending on medical services for the elderly. By the middle of the 1980s, the bioethical discourse increasingly contained debate not only about the rights of the elderly to protection as a vulnerable social group, but also the moral responsibility of the elderly to bear at least part of the cost-containment burden. This strain occurred as part of a broader interest within ethics, and in other areas of political and public discourse, with issues of rationing of health care, priorities, and conceptualizations of justice.[54]

By the late 1980s several explicit proposals concerning the appropriate philosophical bases and justifications for rationing health care to the elderly had been made by some of the leading figures in bioethics.[55] Although controversy surrounded the introduction of some of these proposals—in particular, Callahan's suggestion that chronological age be used as a factor in the denial of treatment to some patients—the door had been opened for development of an area of professional ethical discourse joining the themes of cost containment, rationing, and aging.

In the search for a moral basis for health care rationing, however, there was a general failure to challenge prevailing political definitions concerning the nature and causes of resource scarcity as well as the assumption that these could be alleviated by age-referenced rationing, and little overt attention[56] was being paid to the significant structural inequalities such rationing would exacerbate. These effects are evident in the de facto restriction of the rationing alternative to recipients of publicly financed health care, as in Callahan's quest for limits[57] and the Oregon Health Initiative.

The concept of "rationing" has been readily accepted within bioethical analyses of macro-level health care issues. In a review of four major studies of health care rationing,[58] Reagan notes that "rationing" is used by all of these authors as a mechanism through which to develop ethical principles for health care distribution.[59] Why was the idea of age rationing taken up with such interest in bioethics during the 1980s? One answer may be, as discussed earlier, the turning away from individualism as a singular and transcendent value. Another may be the pessimism many bioethicists who have been directly involved in policy have expressed about the role of their philosophical efforts.[60] The perceived lack of direct influence or authority in the health policy arena may have encouraged some writers (e.g., Daniels, this volume) to develop a theoretical scheme under which age rationing could be justified, while not appearing to support the implementation of such a policy. We suggest further that the philosophical heritage of bioethics may lead its practitioners away from incorporating conflict into theoretical developments, to avoid social conflict within the framework of normative ethics.[61] Ethics has been described as manifesting an internal orientation toward unlimited optimism, in which conflict and oppression cannot fit.[62] Conflict-oriented social power is not a significant element of the normatively defined "good" life or "just" society.

In addition, we suggest that bioethics may be limited to representing a narrow range of values and means-goal motivations, in part due to the narrow range of ethnic, class, and educational experience represented among its practitioners in the United States. However, the extent to which bioethics may represent a socially and structurally relative value system may be obscured by its close association with the positivism of "neutral" scientific thought and disciplinary action structures.[63] The dominant conception of morality within both analytic philosophy and the branch of applied ethics is itself "positivist"—"a consistent, rationally justified system of norms that are applied to the facts of problematic cases to generate resolutions".[64]

The appearance of ideological neutrality in positivist endeavors is a significant element in the legitimation processes of medicalization. Estes and Binney have described the biomedicalization of aging in which aging has come to be understood as a medico-moral social problem.[65] The "bioethicalization" of problems brings them within the realm of a particular professional expertise—that of the professional moral authority. Further, the tendency has been noted within bioethics to maintain a categorical distinction between the social and the ethical[66] so that certain types of "social problems" are removed from moral scrutiny. These processes work together to support a technical-moral construction of conditions, such as the status of the elderly and the societal prospects of an aging society, which have complex social and structural bases. Thus while professional ethicists may perceive that they have no authority,[67] their involvement in the political sphere may be viewed as part of larger defining processes that do have power-related consequences.

An examination of how problems—for example, aging—come to be defined is important because these definitions are likely to become objective reality in one form or another.[68] Specifically, the dominant "definitions of the situation" are likely to become objectified in policy language and implementation.[69] The resultant policies, however, are constructed in ways that embody structural interests, that is, interests that are built into the way our social institutions are organized and operate. Both the definitions and policies tend to *institutionalize* the advantages of some selected groups and professions through the structures created in the policy design and implementation. Structural interests limit the actions that actors in the situation may make.[70] These constraints appear in the form of mandated structural arrangements of agencies and actors that comprise the decision-making network[71] as well as the power and opportunities for information and prestige available to individuals within the social structure.[72] Structural arrangements shape the limits of what is conceivable[73] and the institutionalization of what is "real." Although socially generated, expert opinion and knowledge underlying the policy choices take on the character of objective reality, regardless of inherent validity.[74] As a result, what exists then appears to be both right and inevitable.[75] In this manner the origins of the structural and ideological constructs that are socially engendered and taken as objective reality are lost from collective consciousness, much as the metaphorical origins of much scientific language blend into how we come to know a thing itself.[76]

Conclusion

The formalism and positivism of medical ethics, as well as its connection with the scientific/technological field of medicine, may tend to remove bioethics from scrutiny as a vehicle for values consistent with dominant political structural interests.[77] However, Habermas argues that science and technology, while claiming to be objective and value-neutral, are far from being so.[78] Scientific experts apply their knowledge to the social sphere and help to legitimate decisions made on the behalf of dominant interests. Lay persons, without possession of esoteric knowledge, are effectively barred from decision making. As a result, what may be highly political issues become depoliticized. Following Habermas, bioethical decision making depoliticizes (or treats as apolitical) issues that are key elements of political struggles in the health care policy arena. Kaufert describes how the assertion that an issue is purely medical in nature can be seen as a "tactic" in struggles for (political) control, both at the level of public policy (i.e., who has the right to participate in government decision making) and in patient/physician encounters.[79] Likewise, the assertion that an issue is medico-moral in nature places a conceptual emphasis on an institutionalized interpretation of relevant moral norms and values,[80] and obscures the political nature of a struggle among self-interested parties over power and resources.

The inadequacy of the rational model of behavior within bioethical reasoning on the allocation of societal resources stems from the focus it places on the behavior of the individual, whether consumer or health care provider, rather than the systemic momentum of the health services market. The theoretical foundations of bioethics (libertarianism, utilitarianism, egalitarianism, and contractarianism) deal with action primarily in terms of individual, calculating, isolated, self-interested actors.[81] In the case of many elderly, their behavior as consumers in the face of the market forces bounding their care options has little to do with opportunities for rational choice. This perspective belies the assumption, voiced by Veatch that "Our resources are finite. Our needs, or at least our desires, are infinite."[82] The pool of resources is continually created anew in the pursuit of profit and expansion. The notion of rationality, venerated as it is, ensures the ideological primacy of the market and the justification for state action to bolster private enterprise.

In this essay we have suggested that the tacit acceptance within bioethics of political and economic constructions of reality provides both rationale and moral characterizations of underlying ideological positions, as opposed to challenging, with critical reasoning, the claims of crisis and scarcity that require individual-level sacrifices of life and health. Arguing the merits of competing rationing proposals makes this no less the case. A similar lack of critically reflexive dialogue within American bioethics permits the focusing on a narrow range of values and variables, forcing choices between absolutes and creating the ethical problems that become its subject matter—"Self versus others, body versus mind, individual versus group, public versus private, objective versus subjective, rational versus nonrational, lie versus truth, benefit versus harm, rights versus responsibilities, independence versus dependence, autonomy versus paternalism, liberty versus justice."[83] And, we would add, old versus other.

A relevant and classic historical critique of medical sociology has been offered by Robert Straus.[84] Arguing that there are two medical sociologies—the sociology of medicine and sociology in medicine—Straus contrasts two forms of the uses of social science analysis in the study of the medical/health community. The first, sociology of medicine, refers to the study of the health and medical community from a social science perspective outside of the "house of medicine" and which retains the critical theoretical and empirical criterion that is the standard of disciplinary research. The other, sociology in medicine, refers to work that loses its unique disciplinary perspective due to an uncritical immersion in the assumptions, ideology, and structures of its subject matter.

The field of bioethics is subject to a similar tension in the social construction of its body of knowledge. How can bioethics meaningfully engage the important policy debates of its time while maintaining a critical and objective stance toward the assumptions and ideologies of its subject matter? An important distinction exists between being "critical" of activities and maintaining a critical distance from the systems or structures in which those activities are embedded. The latter position can afford the perspective from which to problematize taken-for-granted constructions of reality.

The continued move in the structure of health care delivery toward managed care and cost-containment measures will ensure that rationing will be an element, and a divisive one, of continuing national, state, and local health policy debates. Ethical justification of rationing must go beyond the service of select common goals if individuals are to be asked to make unique sacrifices to achieve these goals. As the politics of crisis has shown, calls for sacrifice have strategic potential. We suggest, rather, a model of the intergenerational stake to express a more organic image of the complex ties, conflicts, interests, and needs of broadly defined social elements. More critical attention to defining the empirical community may clarify justifications for burden-shifting proposals and lessen the likelihood of co-optation of moral legitimacy by strategic interests.

Thus we conclude with a challenge to the field of bioethics. We call for a critical perspective based on an aggressive and rigorous reflexivity concerning the macro social, cultural, political, and economic issues inherent in the debate on rationing health care for the elderly. This reflexivity must also lead to a new awareness that policy is not outside of the realm of theory but is integral to it.[85] Bioethics is more than a discourse of reason; it is a social formation that plays a role, intentionally or not, in discourses and actions of power. At the very least, the evolving and increasingly complex relationship between bioethics and public policy formulation needs to be better understood.

Notes

1. Bruce Jennings, "Ethics and Ethnography in Neonatal Intensive Care," in George Weisz, ed., *Social Science Perspectives on Medical Ethics* (Philadelphia: University of Pennsylvania Press, 1990), 262.

2. Philip R. Lee and Carroll L. Estes, "Introduction," in Philip R. Lee and Carroll L. Estes, eds., *The Nation's Health*, 4th ed. (Boston: Jones and Bartlett, 1994), xi–xiv.

3. Ibid.

4. Adele Clarke and Theresa Montini, "The Many Faces of RU486: Tales of Situated Knowledges and Technological Contestations," *Science, Technology and Human Values* 18 (1993): 42–78.

5. U.S. Senate, Special Committee on Aging, *The Future of Medicare* (Washington, D.C.: U.S. Government Printing Office, 1983).

6. Anne A. Scitovsky, "Medical Care in the Last Twelve Months of Life: The Relation between Age, Functional Status, and Medical Care Expenditures," *Milbank Memorial Fund Quarterly: Health and Society* 66 (1989): 640–60.

7. Robert H. Binstock, "The Oldest Old and 'Intergenerational Equity,'" in R. M. Suzman, D. P. Willis, and K. G. Manton, eds., *The Oldest Old* (New York: Oxford University Press, 1992), 394–417.

8. Daniel Callahan, *Setting Limits: Medical Goals in an Aging Society* (New York: Simon and Schuster, 1987).

9. Elizabeth A. Binney and Carroll L. Estes, "The Retreat of the State and Its Transfer of Responsibility: The Intergenerational War," *International Journal of Health Services* 18:1 (1988): 83–96.

10. Carroll L. Estes, "The Aging Enterprise Revisited," *The Gerontologist* 33:3 (1993): 292–98.

11. Peter Berger and Thomas Luckmann, *The Social Construction of Reality* (New York: Doubleday, 1966).

12. Carroll L. Estes, Lenore Gerard, Jane S. Zones, and James Swan, *Political Economy, Health, and Aging* (Boston: Little, Brown, 1984).

13. Murray Edelman, *Political Language: Words That Succeed and Policies That Fail* (New York: Academic Press, 1977); Carroll L. Estes, *The Aging Enterprise* (San Francisco: Jossey-Bass, 1979).

14. For example, Antonio Gramsci, *Selections from the Prison Notebooks,* trans. Quintin Hoare and Geoffrey N. Smith (New York: International Publishers, 1971).

15. Barry Hoffmaster, "The Theory and Practice of Applied Ethics," *Dialogue* 30 (1991): 213–34.

16. Acknowledgment of the legitimating potential, or advantage, of a statement of moral principles emanating from the professional bioethics community was made recently by the Clinton administration. A group of bioethicists was assembled to develop for the Health Care Reform Task Force a statement of moral principles underlying the health care reform effort. Co-chair Nancy Dubler wrote of that experience: "The fact that the leadership of the Task Force saw fit to establish such a group, thereby confirming that bioethics is a player in the arena of health policy, was in itself significant"

("Working on the Clinton Administration's Health Care Task Force," *Kennedy Institute of Ethics Journal* 3:4 [1993]: 422.

17. Ibid.; Paul Menzel, "Public Philosophy: Distinction without Authority," *Journal of Medicine and Philosophy* 15:4 (1990): 411–24.

18. Carroll L. Estes, "Austerity and Aging in the United States: 1980 and Beyond," *International Journal of Health Services* 12:4 (1982): 573–84.

19. R. J. Samuelson, "Busting the U.S. Budget: The Costs of an Aging America," *National Journal* 10:7 (1978): 256–60.

20. Carroll L. Estes, "The Reagan Legacy: Privatization, the Welfare State, and Aging in the 1990s," in John Myles and Jill Quadagno, eds., *States, Labor Markets, and the Future of Old-Age Policy* (Philadelphia: Temple University Press, 1991), 59–83.

21. Carroll L. Estes, "Fiscal Austerity and Aging," in Carroll L. Estes, ed., *Fiscal Austerity and Aging: Shifting Governmental Responsibility for the Elderly* (Beverly Hills, Calif.: Sage, 1983), 20.

22. U.S. Senate, Special Committee on Aging, Administration on Aging, and the American Association of Retired Persons, *Aging America: Trends and Projections, 1987–88* (Washington, D.C.: AARP, 1989).

23. Estes et al., *Political Economy, Health, and Aging.*

24. For example, Daniel Callahan, "Autonomy: A Moral Good, Not a Moral Obsession," *Hastings Center Report* 14:5 (1984): 40–42.

25. See the collected papers in *Hastings Center Report* 14 (1984).

26. Willard Gaylin, "Introduction: Autonomy, Paternalism, and Community," *Hastings Center Report* 14:5 (1984): 5.

27. Callahan, "Autonomy," 42.

28. Robert M. Veatch, "Autonomy's Temporary Triumph," *Hastings Center Report* 14:5 (1984): 38.

29. The methodology of much applied ethics has been commented upon from within the field—for example, Stephen Toulmin, "How Medicine Saved the Life of Ethics," in Joseph P. DeMarco and Richard M. Fox, eds., *New Directions in Ethics: The Challenge of Applied Ethics* (London: Routledge and Keagan Paul, 1986), 265–81—and alternative approaches, notably casuistry, have become more prominent: Albert R. Jonsen and Stephen Toulmin, *The Abuse of Casuistry* (Berkeley: University of California Press, 1988); John D. Arras, "Getting Down to Cases: The Revival of Casuistry in Bioethics," *Journal of Medicine and Philosophy* 16 (1990): 29–51.

30. Renee Fox and Judith P. Swazey, "Medical Morality Is Not Bioethics: Medical Ethics in China and the United States," *Perspectives in Biology and Medicine* 27 (Spring 1984): 336–60.

31. Hoffmaster, "Theory and Practice of Applied Ethics."

32. Ibid., 216.

33. Carol Gilligan, "In a Different Voice," in M. Pearsall, ed., *Women and Values* (Belmont, Calif.: Wadsworth, 1986). For arguments see Mary Jane Larrabee, ed., *An Ethic of Care: Feminist and Interdisciplinary Perspectives* (New York: Routledge, 1993).

34. Public Citizen Health Research Group, "Health Costs $817 Billion for 1992; $1.472 Trillion by 1997," *Health Letter* 8:2 (1992): 9–10.

35. John Ehrenreich and Barbara Ehrenreich, *The American Health Empire* (New York: Vintage, 1971); Uwe E. Reinhardt, "Health Insurance for the Nation's Poor," *Health Affairs* 6:1 (1987): 101–22; Victor R. Fuchs, "The Competition Revolution in Health Care," *Health Affairs* 7:3 (1988): 5–24; Carroll L. Estes, Charlene Harrington, and Solomon Davis, "The Medical Industrial Complex," in E. Borgatta and M. Borgatta, eds., *The Encyclopedia of Sociology* (New York: Macmillan, 1992), 1243–54.

36. U.S. Department of Health and Human Services, "National Health Expenditures, 1988," *Health Care Financing Review* 11:4 (1990): 1–41.

37. Carroll L. Estes and Robert A. Alford, "Systemic Crisis and the Nonprofit Sector: Toward a Political Economy of the Nonprofit Health and Social Services," *Theory and Society* 19:2 (1990): 20–35; Jürgen Habermas, *Legitimation Crisis* (Boston: Beacon Press, 1975), 53–54.

38. Helen Darling, "The Role of the Federal Government in Assuring Access to Health Care," *Inquiry* 23 (1986): 286–95; Margaret B. Sulvetta and Katherine Swartz, *The Uninsured and Uncompensated Care: A Chartbook* (Washington, D.C.: National Health Policy Forum, 1986).

39. Estes, "Reagan Legacy," 60.

40. For example, Richard D. Lamm, "Ethical Health Care for the Elderly: Are We Cheating Our Children?" in T. M. Smeeding et al., eds., *Should Medical Care Be Rationed by Age?* (Totowa, N.J.: Rowman and Littlefield, 1987), xi–xv.

41. Anne A. Scitovsky, "The High Cost of Dying: What Does the Data Show?" *Milbank Memorial Fund Quarterly: Health and Society* 62 (1984): 591–608.

42. J. Lubitz and R. Prihoda, "The Uses and Costs of Medicare Services in the Last Two Years of Life," *Health Care Financing Review* 5:3 (1984): 117–31.

43. S. W. Letsch, K. R. Levit, and D. R. Waldo, "National Health Care Expenditures, 1987," *Health Care Financing Review* 10:2 (1988): 109–22.

44. Information in this paragraph comes from Richard A. Rettig, "Medical Innovation Duels Cost Containment," *Health Affairs* 13:3 (Summer 1994): 7–27.

45. Joseph P. Newhouse, "Medical Care Costs: How Much Welfare Loss?" *Journal of Economic Perspectives* 6:3 (1992): 3–21; Newhouse, "An Iconoclastic View of Health Cost Containment" (Supplement), *Health Affairs* 155 (1993).

46. Noralou Roos and Leslie R. Roos, "Small Area Variations, Practice Style, and Quality of Care," in Lee and Estes, eds., *Nation's Health*, 322–32.

47. Ibid., 325.

48. Ibid., 328.

49. Jan Blustein and Theodore R. Marmor, "Cutting Waste by Making Rules: Promises, Pitfalls, and Realistic Prospects," in Lee and Estes, eds., *Nation's Health*, 333–44.

50. Richard W. Momeyer, "Philosophers and the Public Policy Process: Inside, Outside, or Nowhere at All?" *Journal of Medicine and Philosophy* 15:4 (1990): 391–409.

51. Richard A. McCormick, "Bioethics in the Public Forum," *Milbank Memorial Fund Quarterly: Health and Society* 61:1 (1983): 113–26; Mary Warnock, "Moral Thinking and Government Policy: The Warnock Committee on Human Embroyology," *Milbank Memorial Fund Quarterly: Health and Society* 63:3 (1985): 504–22; John Mendeloff, "Politics and Bioethical Commissions: 'Muddling Through' and the 'Slippery Slope,'" *Journal of Health Politics, Policy and Law* 10:1 (1985): 81–92; Baruch A. Brody, "Quality of Scholarship in Bioethics," *Journal of Medicine and Philosophy* 15:2 (1990): 161–78; Frances M. Kamm, "The Philosopher as Insider and Outsider," *Journal of Medicine and Philosophy* 15:4 (1990): 347–74; Momeyer, "Philosophers and the Public Policy Process"; Menzel, "Public Philosophy"; Martin Benjamin, "Philosophical Integrity and Policy Development in Bioethics," *Journal of Medicine and Philosophy* 15:4 (1990): 375–89.

52. Harry R. Moody, *Ethics in an Aging Society* (Baltimore: Johns Hopkins University Press, 1992).

53. Binney and Estes, "Retreat of the State."

54. Moody, *Ethics in an Aging Society*.

55. Callahan, *Setting Limits*; Norman Daniels, *Am I My Parents' Keeper? An Essay on Justice between the Young and the Old* (New York: Oxford University Press, 1987); Robert M. Veatch, "Justice and the Economics of Terminal Illness," *Hastings Center Report* 18:4 (1988): 34–40; Margaret P. Battin, "Choosing the Time to Die: The Ethics and Economics of Suicide in Old Age," in Stuart F. Spicker, Stanley R. Ingman, and Iam R. Lawson, eds., *Ethical Dimensions of Geriatric Care* (Dordrecht: D. Reidel, 1987), 161–89; Larry R. Churchill, *Rationing Health Care in America: Perceptions and Principles of Justice* (Notre Dame: University of Notre Dame Press, 1987); Paul

Menzel, *Strong Medicine: The Ethical Rationing of Health Care* (New York: Oxford University Press, 1990).

56. With some exceptions, e.g., Nancy S. Jecker, "Age-Based Rationing and Women," *Journal of the American Medical Association* 266 (1991): 3012–15.

57. Callahan, *Setting Limits*, 137–38.

58. Robert H. Blank, *Rationing Medicine* (New York: Columbia University Press, 1988); Callahan, *Setting Limits;* Churchill, *Rationing Health Care;* Daniels, *Am I My Parents' Keeper?*

59. Michael Reagan, "Health Care Rationing: A Problem in Ethics and Policy," *Journal of Health Politics, Policy and Law* 14:3 (1989): 627–33.

60. Dubler, "Health Care Task Force."

61. See Moody, *Ethics in an Aging Society.*

62. Timo Airaksinen, *Ethics of Coercion and Authority: A Philosophical Study of Social Life* (Pittsburgh: University of Pittsburgh Press, 1988).

63. Karl Mannheim, *Ideology and Utopia: An Introduction to the Sociology of Knowledge* (New York: Harcourt, Brace and World, 1936); Jürgen Habermas, "Science and Technology as 'Ideology,'" *Toward a Rational Society* (Boston: Beacon Press, 1970); Susan E. Kelly, "The Value Experts: Structure and Consequences of Ethics in Medicine," ms., University of California, San Francisco, 1991.

The complex concept of ideology and its relation to cultural values and political processes is of key importance in this analysis. In the sense in which Mannheim defines the "total conception of ideology," examination of the ideological nature of modern medical ethics involves analysis of both the social conditions of its development and its conceptual apparatus. The latter refers to fundamental thought systems rather than specific thought concepts, and to the form or mode of experiencing and interpreting reality.

Also following from Mannheim's total conception of ideology, examination of the role of modern medical ethics in the structure of policy development focuses on the functional, rather than the psychological, expression of interests. This approach specifically sublimates analysis of individual intent and agency to examination of the role and outcome of ideas in empirical political processes. Such a focus also regards the significance of ideology as the expression of social relations rather than restricting ideology to its relation to material interests.

64. Barry Hoffmaster, "Morality and the Social Sciences," in George Weisz, ed., *Social Science Perspectives on Medical Ethics* (Philadelphia: University of Pennsylvania Press, 1991), 257.

65. Carroll L. Estes and Elizabeth A. Binney, "The Biomedicalization of Aging: Dangers and Dilemmas," *The Gerontologist* 29:5 (1989): 587–96.

66. Renee Fox, "The Evolution of American Bioethics: A Sociological Perspective," in Weisz, ed., *Social Science Perspectives*, 201–17.

67. Menzel, "Public Philosophy."

68. Estes, *Aging Enterprise*; Carroll L. Estes, "Construction of Reality: Problems of Aging," *Journal of Social Issues* 36:2 (1980): 117–32.

69. Estes, *Aging Enterprise*.

70. Ibid.

71. Steven Lukes, *Essays in Social Theory* (London: MacMillan, 1977).

72. A. C. Twaddle and R. M. Hessler, *Sociology of Health* (St. Louis: Mosby, 1977).

73. Lukes, *Essays in Social Theory*.

74. Estes, *Aging Enterprise*, 6.

75. R. Alford, *Health Care Politics* (Chicago: University of Chicago Press, 1976), 7.

76. Scott L. Montgomery, "Codes and Combat in Biomedical Discourse," *Science as Culture* 2 (1991): 341–89.

77. Kelly, *Value Experts*.

78. Habermas, "Science and Technology."

79. Patricia Kaufert, "Ethics, Politics, and Contraception: Canada and the Licensing of Depo-Provera," in Weisz, ed., *Social Science Perspectives*, 121–41.

80. Kelly, *Value Experts*.

81. Churchill, *Rationing Health Care*, 138.

82. Robert M. Veatch, "Finite Resources in a World of Infinite Needs," in Jack D. McCue, ed., *The Medical Cost-Containment Crisis: Fears, Opinions, and Facts* (Ann Arbor: Health Administration Press Perspectives, 1989), 81–96.

83. Fox and Swazey, "Medical Morality," 355.

84. Robert Straus, "The Nature and Status of Medical Sociology," *American Sociological Review* 22 (1957): 200–204.

85. Alvin Gouldner, *The Coming Crisis in Western Sociology* (New York: Basic Books, 1970).

6

Why Now?

The Growing Interest in Limiting the Lifesaving Health Care Resources Available to Elderly People

John F. Kilner

When health care resources appear insufficient to treat all who need them, the solution increasingly proposed is to limit the lifesaving care available to elderly persons.[1] The two authors writing in Part 1 of this book are only the latest in a series of recent writers who advocate or otherwise identify with this approach.[2] National and state surveys also document significant support for age-related allocation criteria.[3]

There is accumulating evidence, in fact, that age criteria already direct many patient selection decisions in the United States.[4] For example, "lifesaving health care"[5] resources such as intensive care, organ transplants, and kidney dialysis have long been allocated on the basis of the age of the patient.[6] Medical studies controlling for physiological differences among patients indicate that even some nonscarce resources tend to be provided on the basis of age.[7]

Proposals for age-based allocation of health care resources are hardly new. For decades they have occasionally appeared even in conservative religious circles.[8] What accounts for the mushrooming interest in such proposals—both the number of supporters and the torrent of criticism in response? To what other cultural developments are these proposals linked, that they should pose such a promise and a threat?

This concluding chapter examines a range of cultural developments in the United States in an attempt to understand better some of the forces underlying the current attention to age-based allocation in health care. Identifying such forces does not constitute a theoretical argument for or against this approach to allocation. An abundance of such ethical analysis has been published elsewhere.[9] Rather, this chapter seeks to explore the larger context in which the ethical debate is occurring in the United States in order to assess the wisdom of pursuing age-based allocation in this context, regardless of its theoretical strengths or weaknesses.

Before launching into this exploration, some clarification of terms is needed. Many people might identify the subject of this book and chapter as "rationing resources for the elderly." There are two problematic terms in this expression: "rationing" and "the elderly."

Casting the discussion in terms of "rationing" is problematic because of the difference between the basic definition of the word and the implicit meanings that it conveys. A typical dictionary definition of "ration" reads something like "to distribute a limited resource." If that were all that the term involved then there would be little debate over whether or not the United States should engage in the rationing of health care. According to this definition, the United States already rations health care along with virtually every other resource. Every governmental budget debate is a reminder that resources are limited and that some way to distribute them must be devised.

"Rationing," however, suggests something much more threatening to many people. As with a similar term, "triage," it conjures up images of crisis situations, such as wartime, that are unusually harsh and presumably temporary.[10] From this perspective, claims proposing that this term accurately describes the current situation are understandably dismissed as untrue, while assertions that a particular form of rationing should be a part of a normal, long-term approach to health care in the United States are appropriately resisted as unthinkable. To avoid subtly biasing the discussion in favor of those who would reject any form of rationing out of hand, the term "allocation" will be adopted in the pages that follow, even though it covers a broader range of distributive approaches than "rationing" does in some people's minds.

The second problematic term noted above is "the elderly." The literature on health care and health policy is filled with such expressions as "the elderly," "the aged," and "the old." This terminology tends to bias one's view of older people because it verbally reduces persons to a single characteristic. If such persons can legitimately be referred to simply as "the elderly," then *prima facie* it can seem legitimate to view them as a reasonably homogeneous group for the purposes of health care allocation decisions. Whether or not such is the case is a matter to be considered, not an assumption to build in from the outset.

A more neutral terminology is therefore required. Ideally, it would be best to adopt language such as "persons who are relatively old," in order to remind ourselves and others that we are talking about beings who are people like everyone else and yet who have a particular distinguishing characteristic in common—one that is relative rather than absolute. Such an expression is awkward to use repeatedly, however, so a compromise is in order. In an attempt to avoid the subtle bias just noted, a generic word such as "person" or "people" will always follow a term such as "elderly" in the pages that follow. (The age range defined by the term "elderly" will be considered later, but most commonly in the United States the term encompasses everyone age sixty-five and older.)

This chapter, then, is devoted to the cultural developments that provide an essential context for considering the wisdom of explicitly limiting, on the basis of age per se, the lifesaving medical resources allocated to elderly people in the United States. The economic, political, religious, and social dimensions of that context will each be examined in turn.

The Economic Context

The most commonly cited reason for limiting the lifesaving resources available to older people is the economic impact of the rapidly growing number of elderly persons in the United States. The percentage of the U.S. population over age sixty-five has grown from less than 2 percent in 1790 to 12.6 percent in 1990, and the percentage continues to increase. Particularly fast-growing are the ranks of the oldest persons—those eighty-five years or older. By 1990 their number in the United States had reached 3.1 million, representing 1.3 percent of the population; moreover, this number is projected to increase by 46 percent in the next decade.[11]

These escalating numbers, particularly of the oldest persons, signal an escalating need for assistance. Those eighty and older have substantially higher rates of illness and disability even when compared only with persons in their seventies and sixties. Moreover, elderly persons who have severe disabilities are more likely to experience chronic disease, to be older and poorer, and to be more dependent than other elderly persons.[12]

The economic burden of the caregiving required is significant. Consider first the private sphere. Seventy percent of the care needed by disabled elderly persons is provided primarily by family and friends. Overall, up to 30 percent of the work force provides care for elderly persons, with nearly 90 percent of caregiving families having only modest means.[13] In the public sphere, meeting the needs of elderly persons now requires a third of the federal budget, with the proportion likely to rise in the future. In fact, projections place deficits in the Medicare program by early next decade at a level comparable with the entire present federal deficit, due in part to a trend toward making expensive lifesaving medical care more available to older persons.[14]

Such economic burdens are widely considered unacceptable. In a recent study, 90 percent of hospital CEOs admit that even "health care rationing" may be necessary in order to ease them. A different study of medical directors found that as the economic urgency of limiting who can receive lifesaving treatments rises, an age criterion for selecting patients will increase in importance more than any other criterion.[15] This mental association of age and cost is an understandable one. As the reasoning goes: health care for elderly persons is costing more and more money, so in order to cut costs it will be necessary to cut back on the health care resources that will be available to them.

However, seven observations challenge this simple economic rationale for age-based allocation of health care:

1. In other societies, similar population and resource trends are observed, though without nearly the same level of alarm. Offsetting demographic trends—for example, reductions in the numbers of other dependent groups, especially children—are readily brought into the equation.[16] Why is the response different in the United States?

2. Health care costs are increasing due to a variety of factors, many of which have no special connection to elderly persons. Why are older people singled out as a group to bear the brunt of cutbacks in lifesaving care?[17]

3. Resource constraints are (for the most part) due to the fact that the sum total of people's various desires exceeds the total of available resources. In a country that spends $3 billion annually on potato chips, for example, why would people consider preventing a certain group of patients from obtaining lifesaving health care to be one of the best ways to save money?[18]

4. Expenditures on costly lifesaving care for elderly persons are actually not very great at present. Most of the resources devoted to them

are not of a lifesaving nature. While there is the distinct possibility that lifesaving expenditures will increase in the future, there are other types of cutbacks that would more certainly provide economic savings.[19] Why is lifesaving care being specially targeted?

5. The demand of elderly people for limited resources can be reduced in a variety of ways. Why is denying lifesaving care to older persons being debated more energetically than, for instance, providing them with an array of basic services that would lessen the likelihood that they would later need more expensive care?[20]

6. There is more to life than economics. Might not the experience of enduring challenges (e.g., sustaining and caring for elderly persons) sometimes contribute more to the strength (character) of a nation than a more profitable balance sheet?[21]

7. When it is claimed, economically speaking, that elderly persons are receiving a "disproportionate share" of health care resources, the question must be raised: "Disproportionate to what?" They are not receiving disproportionately to their medical need (assuming that medical criteria are being equitably applied to all). Why do those concerned about disproportionate shares so readily assume that the appropriate frame of reference for "proportion" is age?

These seven observations/questions suggest that a more complicated economic trend is at work in U.S. culture than simply a concern to reduce health care or other expenditures. There appear to be other reasons for targeting elderly persons in particular for cutbacks. That lifesaving care is at issue even raises the possibility that there is something undesirable about elderly persons per se.[22]

This outlook is attributable, at least in part, to the increasingly utilitarian orientation of U.S. culture.[23] Utilitarianism is an outlook that identifies right actions as those producing the greatest benefits for the greatest number of people. When employed consciously or unconsciously as a means of determining who should receive limited resources, it predisposes one to view people in terms of whatever contributions are valued most highly by the culture, with a bias toward contributions most readily quantifiable and thus comparable.

In the market-driven U.S. culture, economic productivity is at the top of the list. So it is no surprise that older people, who are less likely to be viewed as economically productive, are not highly valued. They are "retired"—or even more comprehensively put, "retirees"—no longer productive in the ways that matter most in contemporary society. Efforts to defend elderly persons by promoting an image of old age as a time of new possibilities and productivity only reinforce this utilitarian perspective: what matters is productivity.[24]

This emphasis on productivity helps explain the culture's preoccupation with youth. It is the time of greatest productivity and thus possibility—a time most worthy of society's attention and protection. Accordingly, elderly people are commonly referred to in terms of either their distance from youth (e.g., "over the hill") or their decline from youth (e.g., their "sunset years").[25]

The preoccupation with youth is further reflected in the way that older people are greatly underrepresented among those featured in every form of media, particularly in advertising. Most companies are reluctant to identify their product with old age. When elderly persons do appear, studies indicate that they are commonly ridiculed as timid and incompetent or demeaned as "greedy geezers" (who consume but do not produce). Given that by the time a child enters kindergarten he or she has watched between 5,000 and 8,000 hours of television, and that a teenager graduating from high school has been bombarded by as many as 350,000 commercial messages, it is not surprising that people in the United States have deep-seated intuitions that youth is what makes life worthwhile.[26] The decision to exclude elderly people from lifesaving health care is a predictable product of this societal preoccupation with youth.

The utilitarian way of thinking that sustains the emphasis on youth and productivity in the United States has been harshly criticized. For instance, comparing everyone's social contribution has been found to be extremely difficult, since everything potentially of benefit to anyone in society must be considered. Utilitarian thinking has also been castigated for its lack of inherent protections against how badly a person or group can be treated if society finds such treatment to be economically beneficial.

However, even if a utilitarian way of thinking were workable and theoretically sound, the question of what should count as a contribution to society remains. The tendency to focus on economic contributions in the United States is rather different from the perspective of some other societies such as the Akamba people of Kenya. Traditionally the Akamba view persons as much more than economic beings. They accord an elderly poor person as much respect as any socially important person. In fact, old age calls forth a unique veneration.[27]

The great deal of respect accorded to old people in Akamba society is intimately bound up with that culture's view of the relationship between the individual and the community. Whereas the utilitarian view common in the United States conceives of the social good atomistically in terms of individual (mainly job-related) contributions summed over the breadth of society, the Akamba view presupposes a social network of interpersonal relations of which one becomes more and more an essential part the older one becomes. The more interwoven a person becomes with others through time, the greater the damage done to the social fabric when that person is torn away by death.

The cultural values surrounding old age lead many Akamba to make decisions about age-related resource allocation that are rather different from those commonly made in the United States. Asked whether an older or a younger man should be saved when there are resources enough for one only, many Akamba medical personnel have argued that even a very old man should be preferred because he "has more responsibilities" and "is a father to many people."[28] The latter expression, though often literally true in the traditionally polygamous Akamba society, here evokes a broader thought. The older man is a leader, a wise counselor, and an inspiring figure worthy of respect within his community.

There are viable alternatives, then, to the economic, individualistic, youth-oriented outlook adopted by many in countries such as the United States. Even relatively "developed" countries—Sweden, for instance—could be cited as examples of places where greater respect for elderly people leads to age criteria (when they exist at all) that are much less restrictive than those in the United States. Moreover, within the United States itself there are subcultures that resist the values undergirding the broader society's outlook on older people.[29]

Proposals to exclude elderly persons from lifesaving resources, then, are not formulated in a cultural vacuum. One important aspect of the context within which they are formulated is economic. If the economic forces at work are less than morally neutral or are unrespectful of cultural diversity, then it is particularly important to be aware of them when assessing the wisdom of a policy that they foster.

The Political Context

A second important dimension of the context conducive to age-based allocation is political. In this arena there are two major tendencies that render age-based allocation particularly plausible. The first is the tendency to assume that the key resource allocation trade-off determining the health care available to elderly persons is that between the lifesaving and non-lifesaving health care resources devoted to older people. The second is the tendency to view elderly people as a single undifferentiated constituency. Both warrant careful consideration.

The trade-off issue can perhaps best be introduced by noting that it rests on a relatively uncontroversial premise. This premise holds that certain aspects of health care for elderly persons—those instrumental to their quality of life—are significantly underemphasized in U.S. society. In one study of health care professionals and executives, 85 percent emphasize this unmet need.[30] Two commonly cited examples of such need are insufficient palliative care (especially pain control) and inadequate long-term care. Since these topics have already been addressed at length in Parts 1 and 2 of this book, particularly in Jecker's chapter on long-term care, they need only briefly be mentioned here.

Sufficient pain control is a major resource allocation issue not because the medication itself is so expensive. Rather, the reason is that understanding what is required to manage particular patients' pain takes not only an investment of time with each patient but also specific training. To date, such training has been deficient in medical education.[31]

Similarly, long-term care is not merely a problem because resources are insufficient to meet present need. Even more significantly, future need will be much greater because of trends in the age composition of the elderly population, the fertility history (i.e., average number of children) of women who will be retiring, and the living arrangements that will be available to elderly people. One recent study[32] has projected these trends (see table 6-1). Since the need for formal long-term care services is most acute for persons who are very old, have no living children, and are living alone, these trends suggest a growing need for long-term care resources.

The need for greater attention to quality-of-life issues, then, is reasonably well established. However, the issue that has particular political significance—the trade-off issue—is another matter. Increasingly, the need for greater resources devoted to palliative and long-term care for elderly persons is being compared with the need they have for acute (high-technology, expensive, lifesaving) care. It is easy to conclude, then, that since elderly persons have a greater need for the former, they must be denied acute (lifesaving) care so that they may receive better palliative and long-term care. Such is the trade-off that must be faced in the harsh

Table 6-1 Trends Underlying Long-Term Care Needs

	1990	2010	2030
Age composition (in millions)			
65–74	18.7	22.1	35.5
75–84	10.1	13.3	22.6
85 or older	3.3	7.6	10.4
Fertility history of women			
Percent childless	14.0	10.6	18.5
Average number of children	2.86	2.49	1.94
Elderly persons living alone			
(in millions)	10.4	5.5	26.2

Source: Derived from Sheila R. Zedlewski and Timothy D. McBride, "The Changing Profile of the Elderly: Effects on Future Long-Term Care Needs and Financing," *Millbank Memorial Fund Quarterly: Health and Society* 70 (Nov. 2, 1992): 247–75. The figures here for the years 2010 and 2030 represent an average between the baseline and optimistic-mortality projections.

political reality of limited resources. This line of reasoning is found explicitly or implicitly not only in Menzel's and Daniels's essays in this book but also in other prominent proposals for age-based allocation of health care resources. Such proposals commonly illustrate the resource choice an individual must make as age-related. It is portrayed as either a choice between lifesaving care at an old age and the same care at a younger age, or a choice between lifesaving and other care at an old age.[33]

While this way of formulating the trade-off issue points directly to the necessity of denying lifesaving health care to elderly people, it is important to bear in mind that this is not the only way that the trade-off issue can be formulated in public policy deliberations. For example, the trade-off could be seen as a choice, for people of all ages, between lifesaving acute care and long-term care—since people at any age may need either one. Access to certain forms of acute care might then have to be limited for persons of all ages. As long as the political question remains "How can Medicare be saved?" the health care resources available to elderly persons will be subject to the amount of resources that can realistically be poured into this single program.[34]

A special characteristic of the U.S. political process is at work here—

the propensity merely to tinker with current approaches rather than re-think and restructure entire systems. One result is that out of all of the relatively industrialized nations of the world (with the exception of South Africa), only the United States lacks a national system to insure the ac-cess of all its citizens to health care. Viewed from this perspective, the more important political trade-off in the United States could be seen as a choice between health care systems.

Alternatively, if lifesaving health care for persons of all ages were deemed important, the trade-off issue might be seen more in terms of how best to use limited resources for long-term care: whether to contin-ue to emphasize the current institutionalization approach or to place much greater emphasis on less expensive but equally effective geriatric foster care or home health aids.[35] If long-term care were still inadequate, the political trade-off between devoting resources to health care versus other sectors of the federal budget might be reconsidered.[36]

How the central political choice is framed, then, has much to do with the appeal of age-based rationing of health care. Formulating the trade-off in a way that implies that if society wants better palliative and long-term care for elderly persons, then older people must forego acute life-saving care, is only one out of a number of reasonable ways that the key choice(s) could be framed. Why this way is increasingly being chosen probably has something to do with the other pivotal matter of political significance mentioned earlier: how the view of elderly persons as a sin-gle, undifferentiated constituency shapes health-related and other public policy decisions.

The tendency to see older people as basically a homogeneous group for public policy purposes in the United States dates back at least to the 1930s, when the Social Security Act was passed. A stream of programs followed—Medicare, the Older Americans Act, special tax breaks and sup-portive services, a National Institute on Aging, and so on. By the mid-1970s the U.S. House of Representatives Select Committee on Aging (us-ing somewhat elastic criteria) was able to count 134 programs for aging persons, which were being overseen by forty-nine congressional commit-tees and subcommittees.[37]

Admittedly, this stream of programs reflected a compassionate view toward elderly persons in need, a view nourished by the religious con-text to be examined shortly. At the same time, however, these programs reflected the perception that elderly people are poor, weak, and helpless—

that old age per se is a social problem that needs special attention. Each new program reinforced the separateness and inferiority of older people.[38] Medicare was the prime example in the health care arena, implicitly identifying the entire population of elderly people as in need of special treatment where the provision of health care resources is concerned.

More recently, though, the material well-being of the elderly population has been changing, in part because of the effectiveness of these age-based programs.[39] Statistically, older people in the United States have become better off than the average citizen. Yet the federal government has not had the resources necessary to accomplish this while attending sufficiently to other national needs. So the government has spent resources it did not have, budget deficits have become commonplace, and the national debt has soared. Pressure has mounted, as a result, for the government to identify targets for major cutbacks. The economic, religious, and social trends identified elsewhere in this chapter have combined with the improved status of many older people to make resources for elderly persons an appealing candidate.

What can easily be overlooked in this change of attitudes toward the level of resources that should be provided for elderly persons is that this latest trend merely reflects the same crucial assumption as did the earlier and opposite trend. Whereas views of how many resources elderly people should receive have changed, what has not changed is the assumption that older persons are essentially a homogeneous group—at least they are sufficiently the same for public policy purposes. Accordingly, proponents of denying elderly people lifesaving health care sometimes explicitly defend their proposals by noting that programs for the elderly, for example, Medicare, have long treated elderly people as a single undifferentiated constituency.[40] In other words, an assessment of the wisdom of age-based allocation in health care must not merely consider what part of the national pie elderly people "deserve." It must also address the assumption that older people should be treated uniformly when resource allocation decisions are made.

This assumption, now deeply established in people's intuitions about how public policy should be formulated, continues to be nourished by the way that the human life span is structured in the United States. In line with the emphasis on economic productivity noted earlier, the life span is commonly viewed in terms of three periods—pre-work (education), work, and post-work (retirement)[41]—in which it seems "natural" to think of all elderly people as being at the same stage of life and having similar needs. Accordingly, until the resource constraints of recent years there has been relatively little difficulty administering Social Security and Medicare in a way quite contrary to their theoretical justification. Although they were theoretically set up to be a mechanism whereby people saved funds during their working years to finance their own health care and other needs in their post-work years, the current population of elderly persons is in fact supported by taxes paid primarily by those still in their working years. Current generations of workers have grown up with the cultural assumption that elderly people warrant special resource allocations.

Whether elderly persons stand to gain resources (as with the inception of Medicare) or lose them (as under more recent age-based allocation proposals), the common theme needing further attention is the appropriateness of viewing elderly people as an undifferentiated group. An extensive amount of recent research has documented the great diversity of the elderly population. Different individuals and even groups (racial, socioeconomic, gender) age differently, such that elderly people constitute one of the most diverse groups in society.[42]

More to the point, the needs of elderly people for lifesaving medical care—and their abilities to benefit from it—are quite diverse. For over a decade studies have indicated that age per se is a poor predictor of the degree to which any particular elderly patient will benefit from treatment.[43] Admittedly, many elderly patients are so physically weakened that they make poor candidates for organ transplantation, intensive care, or even dialysis; but others bear up well in these circumstances.[44] A given elderly person may be in better physical condition to undergo treatment than a younger person. Certain elderly patients also have a strength of mind and heart that make them better candidates for treatment than some patients half their age.[45] So the deeply ingrained public policy assumption that elderly people can legitimately be viewed as an undifferentiated group, particularly where health care is at issue, is extremely problematic.

This being the case, the meaningfulness of a category of "elderly people" defined as all those sixty-five years of age or older would seem open to question. Indeed, in many cultures outside the United States the concept of being old is tied to specific characteristics of people, such as what they are able to do, rather than to age per se.[46] From this perspective the United States appears preoccupied with what some have termed "the facade of chronological age"—a way of categorizing people that appears to reveal much about them but that really reveals little other than the number of years that have elapsed since their birth.[47]

A growing awareness of this problem has recently begun motivating an attempt to narrow the definition of a "truly old person." This narrowing has occurred in two stages. The first involved distinguishing the "young old" from the "old old." (Note the reduction of people to an age-based adjective similar to the reductionist term "the elderly" discussed near the outset of the chapter.) During the early 1980s people increasingly recognized that those aged sixty-five to seventy-four (the "young old") resemble those younger than them more than they do those older than them in certain (e.g., health-related) respects.[48] Then, a second narrowing occurred. Upon closer examination, people began to see that even seventy-five to eighty-four-year-old people often continue to fare well physically. So the need for a group called the "oldest old"—those aged eighty-five and older—was affirmed.[49]

Rather than correcting the problematic assumption—that older people constitute a group sufficiently homogeneous for public policy (especially health care) purposes—these refinements reinforced it. They merely adjusted the number to be placed at the low end of the elderly range, leaving intact (in effect, reaffirming) the notion that there is a meaningful social group called "elderly" people.

Proponents of barring elderly people from receiving lifesaving health care have typically seized upon this refined categorization as a way to distinguish those elderly persons whom they would bar (i.e., the oldest group) from the other, younger elderly people, whom they would not bar. While this distinction renders their proposal more intuitively plausible as public policy than would be a plan to leave sixty-five-year-old people without even simple lifesaving health care, it is important to recognize that the proposal still depends on two assumptions that have been gaining strength over time: (1) the central trade-off is between lifesaving health care for elderly persons and the palliative and long-term care that they also so desperately need, and (2) elderly people (by whatever age definition) are basically a homogeneous group. Both assumptions must be assessed with care.

The Religious Context

Not only are proposals for age-based allocation of health care resources in the United States arising in a specific economic and political context; they are emerging from a particular religious context as well. Of particular significance is the trend toward the exclusion of religious practices and perspectives from public life. It is not that people are no longer personally interested in religion, but that religion is increasingly seen as more of a liability than an asset in formulating public policies to govern as religiously diverse a population as the United States.[50]

One result has been a loss of meaning surrounding aging. Outlooks on aging are frequently rooted in a religious tradition—or even more than one tradition. Consequently, such outlooks become suspect and it becomes preferable publicly to protect the "right" of individuals to find their own meaning. While some will take advantage of this opportunity to conduct their own religious or quasi-religious pilgrimage to search out such meaning, people tend unconsciously to assimilate from their culture the meaning that "should" be ascribed to aging. As many commentators have noted, people in effect "learn" that the current meaning of old age is precisely its lack of substantive meaning.[51] In the absence of such meaning, it is not surprising that a society would consider reining in escalating health care expenditures by cutting back the resources that allow people of an advanced age to continue living.

Traditionally in the United States, religion has helped to give aging meaning by giving people a framework for coping with aging's ambiguity.[52] Although attaining old age is a common hope, being old is seldom relished. But within certain religious frameworks, the downside of aging—weakness and decline—can itself paradoxically become the opportunity for new life. Without such a framework of redeeming possibilities there is a desperate need to deny aging's downside.

Indeed, the image of old age increasingly being fostered in the United States today is one of vitality and productivity, in which weakness—not to mention dying—has no place. In such a context people depend on medical technology to keep decline at bay. Without God or some other religious power available, technology must foster life in the face of death in the only way that it can—by keeping the patient alive.

The desperate overuse of technology that has resulted has predictably ended up prolonging and adding to the suffering associated with the dying process. As this overuse of technology and increased suffering are recognized in the care of elderly people, an understandable response is to want to bar the offending party, the "lifesaving" technology, from any contact with elderly patients. But before this is done it is important to discern whether this abuse of elderly people is the necessary outcome of employing medical technology or results from using that technology in a vacuum of meaning produced by the exclusion of religion from the public sphere.

Although "religion" in the current context refers to the complete range of religious traditions, what primarily has diminished in the United States is the formative influence of Christianity and, to a lesser extent, Judaism. While this influence has often been referred to as "Judeo-Christian," the term is open to criticism as unrepresentative of any actual religious tradition. There are no "Judeo-Christians"; there are Jews and there are Christians. (However, the moral outlook and cultural influence of Judaism has been very similar to that of Christianity since Judaism is largely rooted in a major body of writing that also is foundational to Christianity—commonly referred to as the "Hebrew Bible" or "Old Testament.") So in light of the statistical and cultural prominence of Christianity in the United States, the following analysis will focus on the waning of the Christian religion as a backdrop to the emergence of age-based resource allocation.[53]

A Christian outlook helps give meaning to old age by providing a holistic context that encompasses both strength and weakness, giving and receiving, youth and old age. To be sure, different strands within Christianity have developed these themes to different degrees, but the themes play a significant role in the scriptural writings that have nourished all of Christianity. Strength, in Christian perspective, is defined not so much in terms of physical prowess as in terms of moral character and wisdom. Wisdom in particular is said to reside primarily in older people simply by virtue of their life experience. (However, because it is also a product of righteousness and God's Spirit, it is possible for younger people to have it and older people to lack it.)

Weakness is acknowledged both in physical and nonphysical forms. It, too, becomes an opportunity for elderly persons rather than a liability for them. Just as wisdom calls for respect from others, weakness calls for protection. It also creates a special occasion for people to draw close to God as they experience God's strength and gain a new appreciation for the spiritual reality that transcends the material sphere.[54]

Similarly, giving and receiving are held together in Christian perspective. The weakness accompanying old age, together with the mandate for younger persons to protect elderly people, insures that older people will do plenty of receiving. In Christian perspective, though, older persons have not merely an opportunity but even a responsibility to give as well.

Life is about serving, by the enabling of God, and older people are given special virtues and circumstances for service, as are people of other ages.[55]

Mutual participation in receiving and giving, in fact, become unifying rather than divisive activities. The needs of young and old people to receive vital resources are not pitted against each other. Rather, a lack of resources on the part of some is typically traced to a misappropriation of resources on the part of others. Needy young and old people alike are championed against those who would disadvantage either group. Similarly, there is no fixed hierarchy of giving in which older persons always give to younger or younger persons always give to older. Instead a dynamic community of people with needs fluctuating over time is envisioned, in which parents not only sacrifice for their children, but later those same children sacrifice for their parents.[56]

A society in which such a holistic perspective had significant influence would have been unlikely to deal with resource limitations by excluding elderly people from lifesaving health care. Old age would have held great potential for meaning as a time of strength and new experience in the midst of weakness—a time of giving and receiving. In fact, people would not even have been responsible for devising their own meaning. They would have lived and died within a community whose story—God's story—promised meaning for their final days from the moment their lives began.[57] While this idealized account never described life in the United States with complete accuracy, it suggests the kind of vision whose impact has faded as the influence of Christianity in the public sphere has steadily weakened over time.

Besides giving meaning to old age itself, in the past Christianity has also fostered a particular outlook on the larger context of life and death within which old age is situated. Life, in Christian perspective, is precious and worthy of special care for a variety of reasons. Life is seen as created by God—in fact, people are viewed as created in the image of God. There is something intrinsic to human life that is uniquely related to God. That God should personally take the form of a human being in Jesus Christ also suggests that life is special. The life of Jesus bore consistent testimony to a commitment to life through the prevention of killing and healing of the sick. Moreover, from a Christian vantage point, life is precious not merely because of what it is but also because of what it can become. A splendorous eternal destiny is promised to believers through the death and resurrection of Christ.

From this perspective, death—particularly as portrayed in the formative Christian Scriptures—is the antithesis of life, both in a material and non-material sense. The choice between life and death goes back to the beginning of the human race, when death is portrayed as the result of people choosing to live apart from God, their true source of life. Sickness and death are also identified as antithetical to the reign of God in the ministry and teaching of Jesus; and later biblical writings more explicitly identify death as an "enemy" that will ultimately be destroyed by God.[58]

An outlook that views human life as so special, regardless of a person's particular characteristics or circumstances, is not likely to sanction decisions to leave all persons above a certain age without lifesaving medical care. Similarly, a perspective that sees human death as an evil to be avoided (when that can be done without creating a greater evil) will not be disposed to leaving older (or any) people without such care. As the public influence of such a perspective diminishes, then, it is not surprising to find growing emphasis on a conception of life within which death is "natural" (perhaps even good) and to be chosen by or for elderly people even when resources are available to enable life to continue.[59]

Life and death, however, are not the only issues surrounding old age concerning which the waning impact of Christianity on U.S. culture makes a difference. Other issues relevant to resource allocation for elderly persons include the perspective Christianity offers on those who are vulnerable and those who are female.

Much has already been said concerning the vulnerability of elderly people as they eventually grow weaker and approach death. The Christian and Jewish traditions, particularly in the scriptural writings they hold in common, are outspoken concerning the importance of protecting those who are vulnerable. The call to "justice" is frequently sounded where the distribution of vital resources is concerned. While justice does include the notion of desert—taking responsibility for one's own behavior—notions of equality and need are much more frequently in view. Equality is rooted in the preciousness of every life along with the importance of mutuality in community, and need reflects the unacceptability of some going without the resources they require in order to live. The demands of justice, then, are invoked against the way people commonly value some persons above others even to the point of seriously jeopardizing the well-being of those most easily victimized.[60] Barring any vulnerable group from lifesaving health care is bound to look suspicious from this perspective.

The special relevance of women to age-based health care allocation, on the other hand, may not be as apparent. Nevertheless, statistics reveal that women would bear the brunt of age-based allocation. While the ratio of elderly men to elderly women in 1960 was five to four, older women now outnumber older men three to two. More specifically, of those age sixty-five to seventy-four, 55 percent are women; of those seventy-five to eighty-four, 62 percent are women; of those over eighty-five, 71 percent are women. So if very elderly people are to be barred from lifesaving health care, it is predominantly women who are in view.

If only publicly funded elderly patients are to go without lifesaving care, women are even more disproportionately affected. Elderly women are more likely than elderly men to live in poverty. In fact, 30 percent of women over eighty-five have incomes below the poverty line. Because they live longer than men (current life expectancies are about seventy-nine and seventy-two, respectively), they are more likely to exhaust their resources and less likely to have a spouse to care for them. A specific age cut-off for receiving lifesaving health care, then, will likely be set high enough to ensure a "full life" as life is typically experienced by men—implicitly devaluing the years beyond that point, which are primarily years of women's lives.[61]

One could argue that such victimization, as with the victimization of vulnerable groups discussed earlier, is contrary to the spirit and teaching of Christianity. Christian Scripture identifies the female-male distinction with slave-free and racial distinctions as inappropriate categories used by one group to assert superiority over another. These writings exhort the community to provide special protection and care to older women in particular, who are frequently widows.[62]

However, there is a marked tension between this perspective on victimization and the ways that the Christian church itself has been implicated in the victimization of vulnerable groups and (especially) women.[63] Warrant for such victimization has even been cited in scriptural writings. So whether the waning of the public influence of Christianity is fostering or inhibiting this victimization is difficult to tell.

It would be easy to overlook here the difference between Christianity (at its best) and what is done in the name of Christianity, but the distinction is potentially too important to ignore. Until relatively recently, many people who called themselves Christians supported the institution of slavery. Even the Christian Scriptures say little explicitly against slavery; in fact, some passages have been construed to support it. Nevertheless, there is such a radically egalitarian and liberationist dynamic in the Christian faith and Scriptures that hindsight shows this dynamic to have been at work in various societies for the ultimate release of slaves.

It is possible, though far from certain, that this same egalitarian and liberationist dynamic has done far more to foster current sensitivities concerning the mistreatment of women in U.S. society than is commonly realized. In other words, the waning of this dynamic in the U.S. public arena may mean the weakening of one of the strongest protections against public policies that victimize women, including a policy of age-based health care allocation.

One last feature of Christianity—a feature it shares with other religious traditions—warrants consideration in the face of the waning influence of religion in the public sphere: Christianity's rootedness in history and in particular communities of believers. Christianity is not a set of abstract theories but a lived faith. As an incarnational religion in which God became flesh and lived among unrighteous people, Christianity in particular tends to insist upon attending to the "fallenness" of the world within which actions and policies are carried out. Justice, for example, is not merely a theoretical ideal used to justify practices that make moral sense only in a perfect world. Rather, it is a mandate to address the actual injustices of the present world.[64]

Accordingly, Christianity is not easily compatible with age-based health care allocation proposals whose proponents admit that age-based allocation would be immoral in the world as it now is—that existing social and economic injustices could cause the application of age-based allocation to compound such injustices.[65] While possibly justifiable in some ideal world, age-based allocation of lifesaving health care in the world as it now is would engage people in a particular instance of abandoning elderly people in need and in that sense excluding them from communal care. Such exclusion would constitute a destructive precedent.[66] In the end, elderly people would likely experience the reality of exclusion from treatment more keenly than they would appreciate the theory that lies behind it. With the weakening public influence of Christianity, however, there may well be less impatience with proposals that are not particularly concerned about the unjust setting within which they would have to be implemented.

Not all age-based proposals neglect the social context within which they would have to be implemented. Callahan's proposals, for example, explicitly acknowledge the loss of meaning surrounding old age and attempt to establish a new understanding of aging to fill the void. People are seen as temporal, community-based beings whose social significance and roles change over time. After living a "natural life span" in which their "life possibilities" have been achieved for the most part, the oldest members of society are to make way for younger generations—particularly by no longer asking society to provide life-sustaining health care resources.[67]

While careful discussion of the adequacy of this approach as an alternative to the traditional system of meaning is beyond the scope of this chapter, several observations are in order. First, the very cultural forces that are responsible for undermining the public influence of Christianity are likely to prevent widespread support for the kind of communitarian perspective proposed. Individualism, discussed below as a pervasive characteristic of "the social context," is likely to be a particularly formidable obstacle (compare Menzel's rejection of Callahan's approach on similar grounds in chapter 1 of this volume).

Second, whatever openness there is to a more communitarian perspective is likely to be shaped in a utilitarian direction—which is problematic for all of the reasons delineated earlier here in the analysis of "the economic context." (In fact, Callahan's language itself is already infused with a utilitarian productivity orientation: life-extending care beyond the natural life span is not warranted because everything of significance by that time has been "accomplished" and "achieved.")[68]

Finally, a communitarian vision in which old age has a determinate and dignified state—even if (re)established on a non-Christian basis—does not readily translate into age-based allocation of life-sustaining health care resources. Such a policy emerges only if the vision is tainted by the two major assumptions examined previously here as central to "the political context." At least prima facie, respect for people as people argues against forcing them to forego resources essential to their continued well-being on the basis of some social or economic characteristic such as age. Many individuals may choose to forego such resources under various circumstances, but that is a matter quite different from forcing the end of life on an entire age-based group. Callahan preserves the appearance of choice by advocating that elderly people themselves be allowed to choose whether they would prefer life-sustaining care or better supportive care.[69] But that approach to the trade-off issue inappropriately focuses the burden of society's resource limitations on elderly people.

An alternative communitarian vision, then, is not likely to replace that of Christianity any time soon. To the extent that it does it is likely to have a problematic utilitarian bent, and it will only support age-based resource allocation to the extent that it embraces dubious assumptions in the political sphere.

The Social Context

The examination of the economic, political, and religious contexts above has already highlighted, at least implicitly, much of what should be noted about the social context in which age-based allocation proposals are being debated. However, two areas need further attention in this concluding section: persistent discomfort toward elderly people in U.S. society today and the social trend toward accepting various forms of so-called euthanasia.

Thinly disguised beneath public acclamations of the wonderful possibilities of old age there persists a deep reservoir of discomfort concerning elderly people. This discomfort takes a variety of forms, ranging from distrusting to demeaning and blaming to abusing.

Distrust is evident particularly in the lack of confidence people have that elderly persons can make good decisions. Whereas the decision-making capacity of younger adults is generally taken for granted in the absence of evidence to the contrary, observers have noticed that people often assume that the capacity of older persons is compromised.[70] It is not surprising, then, that government programs for elderly persons have not tended to provide direct income maintenance that would allow older people to make independent choices, but instead have subsidized service providers on their behalf.[71] In such an environment, it is also predictable that elderly people would not be trusted to make wise decisions to forego life-saving treatment when it would not provide significant benefit—hence the rise of age-based health care allocation to make those decisions for them.

The stereotyping, though, is even more demeaning than this. Old age has come to symbolize failure—or worse. In a scientific age with endless possibilities, health is now the norm. Deviations are to be "cured." Aging (not to mention death) constitutes failure because it cannot be undone or avoided. As an obstacle to the ultimate triumph of technology, it can even be seen as an evil.[72] In a society that tends to "blame the victim," it is predictable that responsibility for this evil would be lodged with the one who is aging. Withholding lifesaving care then becomes a justifiable social response. If the problem cannot be solved, at least it can be removed.[73]

That this characterization is not too harsh is suggested by the most explicit form that demeaning of elderly people takes in U.S. society, so-called elder abuse. Abuse of older persons usually takes one or more of three possible forms: physical abuse (violent acts and extreme neglect), financial abuse (theft or misappropriation of valuable property), and psychological abuse (dehumanization to the point that life is threatened). This problem has been well documented.[74] A study of this behavior conducted by the U.S. House Select Committee on Aging has found over a million people subject to such abuse, and only one of every five cases is thought to be reported to authorities. Moreover, the figures have been rising throughout the past decade.[75] The possibility of barring elderly people from receiving lifesaving health care resources, then, arises in a social context where widespread frustration is already being expressed toward older persons.

In addition to variously manifested discomfort toward elderly people there is a second feature of the social context of age-based allocation that warrants further attention: the trend toward accepting various forms of so-called euthanasia. As Battin explains in Part 2 of this book, "euthanasia" means different things to different people.[76] As used in the present chapter, the term refers to actions chosen or rejected based on the intention to end life, whether involving direct suicide (physician-assisted or otherwise), killing patients without their consent, or simply withholding or withdrawing treatment (with or without consent) in order to end life. The term is designed to exclude situations in which treatment is withheld or withdrawn for reasons of medical benefit (i.e., because it cannot stop a death that will occur relatively soon, in many cases with the attendant risk that treatment will instead add to the suffering of the dying process). While the term is probably best avoided for public policy purposes because of its variety of meanings and connotations, here it will serve well to identify the trend toward intentionally ending the lives of certain people.

Acceptance of forgoing treatment has been growing—though studies do not always distinguish actively ending someone's life (e.g., by a lethal injection of potassium chloride), intentionally ending life by forgoing treatment, and forgoing unbeneficial treatment. A U.S. poll, for example, has shown that 70 percent of the population would want to have their life-support systems removed should they lapse into an irreversible coma.[77] As early as 1983, a U.S. presidential commission reflected an emerging national consensus regarding the acceptability of forgoing life-sustaining treatment under certain circumstances.[78] In the years since, studies have appeared documenting the frequency with which patients choose to withdraw from such treatment.[79]

Researchers have also documented lesser but growing support for active intervention to bring about death under certain circumstances. In California, for instance, 68 percent of the people already supported such active intervention in 1983 (as compared with 94 percent in support of allowing treatment refusal at the time).[80] More recent polls show similar figures.[81] Nationwide support in the United States for terminating life in some situations appears to run closer to 50 to 60 percent according to public opinion polls.[82] The broad interest in this issue was underscored when the how-to manual on suicide, *Final Exit*, quickly vaulted to the top of the *New York Times* bestseller list in 1991.

Medical opinion seems to be more cautious, as indicated by the controversies in medical circles stirred up by published reports of medically induced deaths and announcements of medical devices to enable patients to commit suicide.[83] Nevertheless, at least one prestigious medical panel has concluded that physician assistance of patients in committing suicide "is certainly not rare" and is to be commended in some circumstances.[84] Surveys of physicians in such locations as Colorado and San Francisco have found about two-thirds of those questioned favoring the option of intentionally ending a patient's life in some situations.[85]

Many life-ending decisions concern the lives of older persons. Moreover, during the 1980s the suicide rate of elderly people (which was already higher than that of other age groups) increased at a greater rate than that of other groups.[86] According to anthropological studies, hastening the deaths of elderly people has traditionally tended to occur only in societies characterized as "simple—hunting and gathering, pastoral and shifting horticultural."[87] In other words, what is occurring in the economically complex United States today is the product of relatively recent cultural forces at work in this society.

Primary among these forces appear to be the lack of control and support people are experiencing regarding decisions that shape their lives. Whereas decisions to end the lives of elderly persons in societies around the world have typically been the product of open discussions involving those persons with their families, in the United States today it is often unclear who is to decide—children, spouses, patients, medical staff, courts of law, or some combination.[88] The assumption in a culture as individualistic as the United States, with its emphasis on personal rights and liberties, is that elderly patients ought to be making the decisions on which their lives depend.[89] However, without the support of family or community, older patients may not easily make decisions—leaving others to step into the vacuum—or may make fatal decisions that would have been different had they had the communal support they needed to go on living. The suicide machine becomes the perfect symbol of the ultimate "quick fix" in a fast-food society that depends on a technological solution for every problem.

The quick fix is as attractive on a societal level as it is on a personal level. If older people can be allowed—even encouraged—to end their lives, then there is no need for an individualistic, utilitarian society to do the much harder work of finding ways to build community and take responsibility for even the least valuable (i.e., the least economically productive) of its members. In such an environment, excluding elderly people from lifesaving care understandably begins to look quite appealing. If social forces are pushing toward allowing or even encouraging older people to die, it hardly makes sense to pay for technology that will prolong their living. At a time when the federal government, through reimbursement mechanisms, is increasingly controlling how much health care is given to whom, refusing to reimburse caregivers for providing lifesaving care to elderly patients (if not barring it altogether) becomes quite conceivable.[90]

Needless to say, "conceivable" or "understandable" does not mean "desirable" or "right." It may well be the case that age-based allocation of lifesaving health care flows predictably from an individualistic social context that demeans elderly people in its search for a quick fix. It is just as understandable that age-based allocation would gain support in a religious context where the waning of Christianity has weakened the impetus to protect the vulnerable and has clouded the meaning and significance of growing old. It is no less surprising that a political context blind to differences among elderly persons and unwilling to tackle simultaneously their most pressing needs would spawn proposals for age-based allocation. And it may also be true that a financially beleaguered economic context infused with utilitarian values readily fosters excluding older people from lifesaving health care. Nevertheless, these trends are not neces-sarily healthy ones; they may instead be cause for alarm.

Public policy formulation needs to attend to more than theoretical ar-guments about the potential justifiability of age-related health care allo-cation. It must also examine the broader cultural context within which such allocation takes place. In light of that context, at least, the wisdom of limiting the lifesaving health care resources available to elderly people is open to serious question.

Notes

1. For an expanded analysis of age-based allocation of health care resourc-es—especially the ethical issues that it raises—see John F. Kilner, *Life on the Line: Ethics, Aging, Ending Patients' Lives, and Allocating Vital Resources* (Grand Rapids: Eerdmans, 1992). The author appreciates permission to draw on that material for several arguments made here.

2. For example, see also Daniel Callahan, *Setting Limits: Medical Goals in an Aging Society* (New York: Simon and Schuster, 1987); Robert M. Veatch, "Distributive Justice and the Allocation of Technological Resources to the Elderly," contract report prepared for the U.S. Congress Office of Technolo-gy Assessment, Washington, D.C., Dec. 1985. Menzel's and Daniels's chap-ters in the present book are included in this stream of writings only because they themselves choose to identify their approaches as related to consider-ations of age. In substance, though, their approaches ultimately are not. Given a choice between age factors and length/quality of benefit factors, Menzel al-ways favors the latter. Similarly, Daniels admits that age-based rationing is likely in practice not to be the result of adopting his Prudential Lifespan Ac-count. So the mere self-characterization of their approaches as open to age-related rationing makes them vulnerable to the cultural critique in the pages that follow.

3. One national survey reported that 35 percent of the respondents sup-ported age criteria and 58 percent opposed them (Pacific Presbyterian Med-ical Center, "Who Lives, Who Dies, Who Decides? National Poll Results," San Francisco, 1987). Another national survey reported that 57 percent of the respondents supported them (Roger W. Evans and Diane L. Manninen, "Pub-lic Opinion concerning Organ Donation, Procurement, and Distribution," results of a survey conducted for the United Network for Organ Sharing by Battelle Human Affairs Research Centers, Seattle, 1987; partially published in *Transplantation Proceedings* 20 [Oct. 1988]: 781–85). One state survey re-ported 19 percent in support and 57 percent opposed (California Health

Decisions, "Preliminary Analysis—Small Group Meetings" [Tustin: California Health Decisions, 1986]); another reported 40 percent in support and 43 percent opposed (Washington Health Choices, *Executive Report* [Seattle: Puget Sound Health Systems Agency, 1986]).

4. For studies of health care professionals, see John F. Kilner, "Selecting Patients When Resources Are Limited: A Study of U.S. Medical Directors of Kidney Dialysis and Transplantation Facilities," *American Journal of Public Health* 78 (Feb. 1988): 144–47; John F. Kilner, *Who Lives? Who Dies? Ethical Criteria in Patient Selection* (New Haven: Yale University Press, 1990); Nora C. O'Malley, "Age-Based Rationing of Health Care: A Descriptive Study of Professional Attitudes," *Health Care Management Review* 16 (Winter 1991): 83–93. See also William R. Hendee, "Rationing Health Care," in James Hamner III and Barbara Jacobs, eds., *Life and Death Issues* (Knoxville: University of Tennessee Press, 1986), 1–10; Joseph Meissner, "Legal Services and Medical Treatment for Poor People: A Need for Advocacy," *Issues in Law and Medicine* 2 (July 1986): 3–13; Basile J. Uddo, "The Withdrawal or Refusal of Food and Hydration as Age Discrimination: Some Possibilities," *Issues in Law and Medicine* 2 (July 1986): 39–59.

5. The term "lifesaving" will be used in this chapter in relation to various chronic as well as acute interventions for two reasons. Not only is the term more familiar than alternatives such as "life-sustaining," but it emphasizes that the alternative to the treatments under consideration is death. "Health care" will also be used here interchangeably with "medical," in that trade-offs between medical and other health care resources will be at issue. It remains true, though, as Estes, Kelly, and Binney note in the previous chapter, that the exclusive reference to "health care resources" in much of the literature, when only "expensive, high-technology, medical resources" are in view, tends to mask the important fact that many of the health care resources needed most by elderly persons are of a different sort (e.g., preventive, palliative, and long-term care).

6. On intensive care, see Jeremiah A. Barondess et al., "Clinical Decision-Making in Catastrophic Situations: The Relevance of Age," *Journal of American Geriatrics Society* 36 (Oct. 1988): 919–37; Donna K. McClish et al., "The Impact of Age on Utilization of Intensive Care Resources," *Journal of the American Geriatrics Society* 35 (Nov. 1987): 983–88; Mary E. Charlson et al., "Resuscitation: How Do We Decide?" *Journal of the American Medical Association* 255 (Mar. 14, 1986): 1316–22; Anne A. Scitovsky, "Medical Care Expenditures in the Last Twelve Months of Life," Final Report to the John A. Hartford Foundation, Mar. 1986.

Regarding kidney dialysis and organ transplantation, see Carl M. Kjellstrand and George M. Logan, "Racial, Sexual, and Age Inequalities in Chronic Dialysis," *Nephron* 45 (1987): 257–63; David A. Ogden, "Organ Procurement and Transplantation," in Gary Anderson and Valerie Glesnes-Anderson, eds., *Health Care Clinics* (Rockville, Md.: Aspen, 1987): 91–108; Jeanie S. Kayser-Jones, "Distributive Justice and the Treatment of Acute Illness in Nursing Homes," *Social Science and Medicine* 23 (Nov. 12, 1986): 1279–86; Roger W. Evans, "Health Care Technology and the Inevitability of Resource Allocation and Rationing Decisions," *Journal of the American Medical Association* (Apr. 15–29, 1983): 2047–53, 2208–19.

On heart transplantation specifically, see *National Heart Transplantation Study* (Seattle: Battelle Human Affairs Research Centers, 1984); Roger W. Evans and Junichi Yagi, "Social and Medical Considerations Affecting Selection of Transplant Recipients: The Case of Heart Transplantation," in Dale H. Cowan, ed., *Human Organ Transplantation* (Ann Arbor: Health Administration Press, 1987), 27, 29. The difficulty of obtaining a heart transplant for those over fifty is one of the main reasons pioneer artificial heart recipients Barney Clark and William Schroeder wanted the new device. The upper age limit then being placed upon artificial heart recipients was sixty-five. See Timothy M. Smeeding, "Artificial Organs, Transplants, and Long-Term Care for the Elderly: What's Covered? Who Pays?" in Timothy M. Smeeding, ed., *Should Medical Care Be Rationed by Age?* (Totowa, N.J.: Rowman and Littlefield, 1987), 144; William C. DeVries et al., "Clinical Use of the Total Artificial Heart," *New England Journal of Medicine* 310 (Feb. 2, 1984): 278; Otto Friedrich, "One Miracle, Many Doubts," *Time*, Dec. 10, 1984, 73. Concerning the use of age criteria in the treatment of heart disease generally, see Craig Fleming et al., "Is Coronary-Care-Unit Admission Restricted for Elderly Patients? A Multicenter Study," *American Journal of Public Health* 81 (Sept. 1991): 1121–26.

7. Regarding treatment of breast cancer, see Sheldon Greenfield et al., "Patterns of Care Related to Age of Breast Cancer Patients," *Journal of the American Medical Association* 257 (May 22–29, 1987): 2766–70. Cf. Jonathan Samet et al., "Choice of Cancer Therapy Varies with Age of Patient," *Journal of the American Medical Association* 255 (June 27, 1986): 3385–90; Terrie Wetle, "Age as a Risk Factor for Inadequate Treatment," *Journal of the American Medical Association* 258 (July 24–31, 1987): 516. Regarding treatment of acute illnesses, see Kayser-Jones, "Distributive Justice."

8. For example, see Norman Anderson, *Issues of Life and Death* (Downers Grove, Ill.: InterVarsity Press, 1976), 102, drawing on the work of G. R. Dunstan, *The Artifice of Ethics* (London: SCM Press, 1974), 89ff.

9. For survey articles, see John F. Kilner, "Age Criteria in Medicine: Are the

Medical Justifications Ethical?" *Archives of Internal Medicine* 149 (Oct. 1989): 2343–46; Kilner, "Age as a Basis for Allocating Lifesaving Medical Resources: An Ethical Analysis," *Journal of Health Politics, Policy and Law* 13 (Fall 1988): 405–23; Nancy S. Jecker and Robert A. Pearlman, "Ethical Constraints of Rationing Medical Care by Age," *Journal of the American Geriatric Society* 37 (Nov. 1989): 1067–75. For book-length treatments, see Harry R. Moody, *Ethics in an Aging Society* (Baltimore: Johns Hopkins University Press, 1992); Robert L. Barry and Gerard Bradley, eds., *Set No Limits: A Rebuttal to Daniel Callahan's Proposal to Limit Health Care for the Elderly* (Urbana: University of Illinois Press, 1991); Robert H. Binstock and Stephen G. Post, "Old Age and the Rationing of Health Care," in Robert H. Binstock and Stephen G. Post, eds., *Too Old for Health Care?* (Baltimore: Johns Hopkins University Press, 1991), 1–12; Nancy S. Jecker, ed., *Aging and Ethics* (Clifton, N.J.: Humana Press, 1991); Paul Homer and Martha Holstein, eds., *A Good Old Age?* (New York: Simon and Schuster, 1990); James Thornton and Earl Winkler, eds., *Ethics and Aging* (Vancouver: University of British Columbia Press, 1988); and Smeeding, *Should Medical Care Be Rationed by Age?*

10. Problems with the term "rationing" are discussed in Moody, *Ethics in an Aging Society,* 198–206; Charles J. Dougherty, "Ethical Problems in Healthcare Rationing," *Health Progress* 72 (Oct. 1991): 32–34; Larry R. Churchill, *Rationing Health Care in America: Perceptions and Principles of Justice* (Notre Dame: University of Notre Dame Press, 1987), 5–19; Ruth Macklin, "Ethical Problems in Rationing Medical Care," *Infection Control* 6 (Sept. 1985): 375–76; Mary A. Baily, "Rationing and American Health Policy," *Journal of Health Politics, Policy, and Law* 9 (Fall 1984): 489–501. On the concept of "triage," see George P. Smith, "Triage: Endgame Realities," *Journal of Contemporary Health Law and Policy* 1 (Spring 1985): 143–51; James F. Childress, "Triage in Neonatal Intensive Care: The Limits of Metaphor," *Virginia Law Review* 669 (Apr. 1983): 547–61; Gerald R. Winslow, *Triage and Justice* (Berkeley: University of California Press, 1982), 1–11; Douglas A. Rund and Tondra S. Rausch, *Triage* (St. Louis: C. V. Mosby, 1981); Nora K. Bell, "Triage in Medical Practices: An Unacceptable Model?" *Social Science and Medicine* 15F (Dec. 1981): 151–56.

11. Jane A. Boyajian, "Sacrificing the Old and Other Health Care Goals," in Jecker, ed., *Aging and Ethics,* 320.

12. Binstock and Post, "Old Age," 7–8; Boyajian, "Sacrificing the Old," 320.

13. Commonwealth Fund Commission on Long-Term Care Assistance, "Help at Home: Long-Term Care Assistance for Impaired Elderly People" (Baltimore: Commonwealth Fund, 1989); Boyajian, "Sacrificing the Old," 320.

14. Moody, *Ethics in an Aging Society,* 5; Daniel Callahan, "Afterword:

Daniel Callahan Responds to His Critics," in Homer and Holstein, eds., *A Good Old Age?* 304–6; Henry J. Aaron et al., *Can America Afford to Get Old?* (Washington, D.C.: Brookings Institution, 1989); Michael Hosking et al., "Outcomes of Surgery in Patients 90 Years of Age and Older," *Journal of the American Medical Association* 261 (Apr. 7, 1989): 1909–15; Henry L. Edmunds et al., "Open-Heart Surgery in Octogenarians," *New England Journal of Medicine* 319 (July 21, 1988): 131–36; Gregory De Lissovoy, "Medicare and Heart Transplants: Will Lightning Strike Twice?" *Health Affairs* 7 (Winter 1988): 61–72; John Holahan and John L. Palmer, "Medicare's Fiscal Problems: An Imperative for Reform," *Journal of Health Politics, Policy, and Law* 13 (Spring 1988): 53–81.

15. "CEOs Polled See Health Care Rationing as a Future Possibility," *AHA News* 28 (June 1992): 3; Kilner, "Selecting Patients."

16. See, for example, Robert L. Kane and Rosalie A. Kane, *A Will and a Way* (New York: Columbia University Press, 1985), 256.

17. For further probing of this question, see Robert H. Binstock, "Another Form of Elderly Bashing," *Journal of Health Politics, Policy, and Law* 17 (Summer 1992): 271; Binstock, "Aging and the Politics of Health-Care Reform," in Carl Eisdorfer et al. eds., *Caring for the Elderly* (Baltimore: Johns Hopkins University Press, 1989), 434; Binstock, "The Oldest Old: A Fresh Perspective or Compassionate Ageism Revisited?" *Milbank Memorial Fund Quarterly: Health and Society* 63 (Spring 1985): 433; Binstock and Post, "Old Age and the Rationing of Health Care," 4; Lawrence DeBrock, "Efficient Allocation of Health Care to the Elderly," in Barry and Bradley, eds., *Set No Limits,* 93–115; Eike-Henner W. Kluge, "The Calculus of Discrimination: Discriminatory Resource Allocation for an Aging Population," in Thornton and Winkler, eds., *Ethics and Aging,* 95.

18. Christine K. Cassel, "The Limits of Setting Limits," in Homer and Holstein, eds., *A Good Old Age?* 200; Nancy B. Cummings, "Social, Ethical, and Legal Issues Involved in Chronic Maintenance Dialysis," in John Maher, ed., *Replacement of Renal Function by Dialysis,* 3d ed. (Boston: Kluwer, 1989), 1141; Eli Ginzberg, "How to Think about Health-Care for the Elderly," in Eisdorfer et al., eds., *Caring for the Elderly,* 459.

19. Dennis W. Jahnigen and Robert H. Binstock, "Economic and Clinical Realities: Health Care for Elderly People," in Binstock and Post, eds., *Too Old for Health Care?* 13–43; Binstock and Post, "Old Age and the Rationing of Health Care," 6–7; David C. Thomasma, "From Ageism toward Autonomy," in Binstock and Post, eds., *Too Old for Health Care?* 145.

20. Cf. Ginzberg, "How to Think," 465.

21. Cf. Christine K. Cassel and Bernice L. Neugarten, "The Goals of Med-

icine in an Aging Society," in Binstock and Post, eds., *Too Old for Health Care?* 88.

22. Needless to say, there are a host of other reasons given by proponents of age-based allocation for limiting lifesaving care. The point here is not that the "real reason" is something different, but that there are forces at work in the culture that may well make the reasons offered more intuitively attractive (or less offensive) than they would otherwise seem on their own merits.

23. Regarding this increasing orientation, see Robert P. George, "Life as an Evil; Death as a Good: Dualism and Callahan's Inversion," in Barry and Bradley, eds., *Set No Limits*, 18; Terrie Wetle, "Ethical Issues and Value Conflicts in Geriatric Care," in Eisdorfer et al., eds., *Caring for the Elderly*, 410; George P. Smith, "Death Be Not Proud: Medical, Ethical, and Legal Dilemmas in Resource Allocation," *Journal of Contemporary Health Law and Policy* 1 (Spring 1987): 50–51; Don S. Browning, "Hospital Chaplaincy as Public Ministry," *Second Opinion* 1 (1986): 73; Mark Siegler, "Should Age Be a Criterion in Health Care?" *Hastings Center Report* 14 (Oct. 1984): 25; John F. Kilner, "Who Shall Be Saved? An African Answer," *Hastings Center Report* 14 (June 1984): 19–21; Richard B. Brandt, "The Real and Alleged Problem of Utilitarianism," *Hastings Center Report* 13 (Apr. 1983): 37–43; Winslow, *Triage and Justice,* 22; Rashi Fein, "What Is Wrong with the Language of Medicine?" *New England Journal of Medicine* 306 (Apr. 1982): 863.

24. Cassel and Neugarten, "Goals of Medicine," 83; Thomas H. Murray, "Meaning, Aging, and Public Policy," in Binstock and Post, eds., *Too Old for Health Care?* 165, 171; Henry C. Simmons, "Countering Cultural Metaphors of Aging," *Journal of Religious Gerontology* 7:1–2 (1990): 156; Thomas R. Cole, "The Specter of Old Age: History, Politics, and Culture in an Aging America," *Tikkun* 3 (Sept.–Oct. 1988): 18; David J. Maitland, *Aging: A Time for New Learning* (Atlanta: John Knox Press, 1987), 2ff.; J. Gordon Harris, *God and the Elderly* (Philadelphia: Fortress Press, 1987), 110; Victoria Secunda, *By Youth Possessed: The Denial of Age in America* (Indianapolis: Bobbs-Merrill, 1984), 52. For an analysis of the history of U.S. culture's preoccupation with economic productivity, see Thomas R. Cole, "The 'Enlightened' View of Aging: Victorian Morality in a New Key," *Hastings Center Report* 13 (June 1983): 34–30.

25. Simmons, "Countering Cultural Metaphors," 155–59; Emily Friedman, "Health Care's Changing Face: The Demographics of the 21st Century," *Hospitals* 65 (Apr. 1991): 37.

26. Secunda, *By Youth Possessed,* 54–75; in Binstock and Post, "Old Age and the Rationing of Health Care," 3.

27. Joseph Muthiani, *Akamba from Within: Egalitarianism in Social Rela-*

tions (New York: Exposition Press, 1973), 74; Kivuto Ndeti, *Elements of Akamban Life* (Nairobi: East Africa Publishing House, 1972), 68–69; John S. Mbiti, *Concepts of God in Africa* (London: S.P.C.K., 1970), 207. Western influences, though, are now altering the traditional Akamba view somewhat. See Kilner, "Who Shall Be Saved?"

28. Kilner, "Who Shall Be Saved?" The expressions here are taken from the interviews with Kiua Mulela (Muvuti Location) and Esther Nthenya (Mbiuni Location).

29. Regarding other countries, see Howard Brody, *Ethical Decisions in Medicine*, 2d ed. (Boston: Little, Brown, 1981), 225; Ramon Velaz et al., "Treatment of End-Stage Renal Disease," *New England Journal of Medicine* 5 (Feb. 1981): 356. On U.S. subcultures, see Stephen G. Post, "Justice for Elderly People in Jewish and Christian Thought," in Binstock and Post, eds., *Too Old for Health Care?* 129.

30. O'Malley, "Age-Based Rationing."

31. Kathleen M. Foley, "The Relationship of Pain and Symptom Management to Patient Requests for Physician-Assisted Suicide," *Journal of Pain and Symptom Management* 6 (July 1991): 289–97; Richard A. McCormick, "Physician-Assisted Suicide: Flight from Compassion," *Christian Century* 4 (Dec. 1991): 1133.

32. Sheila R. Zedlewski and Timothy D. McBride, "The Changing Profile of the Elderly: Effects on Future Long-Term Care Needs and Financing," *Milbank Memorial Fund Quarterly: Health and Society* 70 (Nov. 2, 1992): 247–75, employ the DYNASIM computer model to generate these projections.

33. For example, see Menzel's first major example (in his essay in this volume), which features choices categorized by three age brackets: thirty to fifty, fifty to seventy, and over seventy. Similarly, see Daniels's first illustration of the typical person (in his essay in this volume): "I must," he says, "be willing to trade coverage for some [health care] needs at certain stages of my life for coverage at others." Cf. Callahan, "Afterword," 300–301. This outlook is also reflected at the outset of Jecker's defense of long-term care (in her essay in this volume), where she suggests that older people need long-term care rather than lifesaving care.

34. Cf. Binstock, "Oldest Old," 443; Kane and Kane, *A Will and a Way*, 256–57.

35. O'Malley, "Age-Based Rationing," 85, 91; Mary T. Koska, "Alternative Care: Aide Shortage Limits Home Health Delivery," *Hospitals* 62 (May 5, 1988): 63; Kathryn L. Braun and Charles L. Rose, "The Hawaii Geriatric Foster Care Experiment: Impact Evaluation and Cost Analysis," *The Gerontologist* 26 (Oct. 1986): 516–24.

36. In fact, Kane and Kane (*A Will and a Way*, 259–60) even question the assumption that long-term care should be treated as part of the health care budget, since it involves so much more than is generally considered to be health care.

37. Binstock and Post, "Old Age and the Rationing of Health Care," 1–2; Binstock, "Aging and the Politics of Health-Care Reform," 428–29; Moody, *Ethics in an Aging Society*, 6; U.S. House of Representatives, Select Committee on Aging, *Federal Responsibility to the Elderly: Executive Programs and Legislative Jurisdiction* (Washington, D.C.: U.S. Government Printing Office, 1976).

38. For different slants on this theme, see Thomas R. Cole, *The Journey of Life* (New York: Cambridge University Press, 1992), 237; K. Brynolf Lyon, *Toward a Practical Theology of Aging* (Philadelphia: Fortress Press, 1985), 28; Secunda, *By Youth Possessed*, 52.

39. For a more detailed analysis, see Binstock and Post, "Old Age and the Rationing of Health Care," 2–3; Binstock, "Aging and the Politics of Health-Care Reform," 433–34; Cole, "Specter of Old Age," 14.

40. For example, see Callahan, "Afterword," 315.

41. See Cole, "Specter of Old Age," 17.

42. Entire collections of articles, such as Scott A. Bass et al., *Diversity in Aging* (Glenview, Ill.: Scott Foresman, 1990), document this feature of growing old. See also Cassel and Neugarten, "Goals of Medicine," 79; Nancy S. Jecker, "Appeals to Nature in Theories of Age-Group Justice," in Nancy Jecker, ed., *Aging and Ethics* (Clifton, N.J.: Humana Press, 1991), 279–81; Cassel, "Limits of Setting Limits," 202–3; Linda K. George, "Social Participation in Later Life: Black-White Differences," in James Jackson, ed., *The Black American Elderly* (New York: Springer, 1988), 102.

43. For example, Jahnigen and Binstock, "Economic and Clinical Realities," 13–43; Nathan W. Shock et al., *Normal Human Aging: The Baltimore Longitudinal Study of Aging* (Washington, D.C.: U.S. Government Printing Office, 1984); James F. Fries and Lawrance M. Crapo, *Vitality and Aging: Implications of the Rectangular Curve* (San Francisco: W. H. Freeman, 1981). These and similar studies are discussed in Thomasma, "From Ageism toward Autonomy," 145; Cassel and Neugarten, "Goals of Medicine," 79; Binstock and Post, "Old Age and the Rationing of Health Care," 7; Arnold Arluke and John Peterson, "Accidental Medicalization of Old Age and Its Social Implications," in Christine L. Fry et al., eds., *Aging Culture and Health* (Westport, Conn.: Praeger, 1981), 276–77.

44. John D. Pirsch et al., "Orthotopic Liver Transplantation in Patients 60 Years of Age and Older," *Transplantation* 51 (1991): 431–33; Thomas E. Starzl

et al., "Liver Transplantation in Older Patients," *New England Journal of Medicine* 19 (Feb. 1987): 484; Evans and Yagi, "Social and Medical Considerations," 29; L. Westlie et al., "Mortality, Morbidity, and Life Satisfaction in the Very Old Dialysis Patient," *Transactions of the American Society for Artificial Internal Organs* 30 (1984): 21–30; Tom A. Hutchinson et al., "Predicting Survival in Adults with End-Stage Renal Disease: An Equivalence Index," *Annals of Internal Medicine* 96 (April 1982): 417–23.

45. J. Grimley Evans, "Age and Equality," *Annals of the New York Academy of Sciences* 530 (1988): 120; Hastings Center, *Guidelines on the Termination of Life-Sustaining Treatment and the Care of the Dying* (Briarcliff Manor, N.Y.: Hastings Center, 1987), 136; Wetle, "Age as a Risk Factor," 516; Arthur L. Caplan, "Equity in the Selection of Recipients for Cardiac Transplants," *Circulation* 75 (Jan. 1987): 16; Patricia M. McKevitt et al., "The Elderly on Dialysis: Physical and Psychosocial Functioning," *Dialysis and Transplantation* 15 (Mar. 1986): 135.

46. Kilner, "Who Shall Be Saved?"; Lowell D. Holmes, "Anthropology and Age: An Assessment," in Christine Fry et al., eds., *Aging in Culture and Society: Comparative Viewpoints and Strategies* (New York: Praeger, 1980), 277.

47. See Lyon, *Practical Theology of Aging,* 29, and sources cited therein.

48. For example, see Fleming et al., "Coronary-Care Unit Admission," 1123; Ginzberg, "How to Think," 451; Binstock, "Aging and the Politics of Health-Care Reform," 431.

49. This development is discussed in Binstock, "Oldest Old," 423–427; Binstock, "Aging and the Politics of Health-Care Reform," 432.

50. For further elaboration and documentation of this development, see John M. Cuddihy, "Perspective: Why Are We Afraid to Talk about God?" *Second Opinion* 17 (July 1991): 118–23.

51. See Lyon, *Practical Theology of Aging,* 22, 29; Stanley Hauerwas, "The Limits of Medicine," in Homer and Holstein, eds., *A Good Old Age?* 122–23; Daniel Callahan, "Can Old Age Be Given a Public Meaning?" *Second Opinion* 15 (Nov. 1990): 21; John H. Weston, "Aging the Last Stage? or, The Drama Continued?" *Second Opinion* 16 (Mar. 1991): 123.

52. Lyon, *Practical Theology of Aging,* 19; Cole, "Specter of Old Age," 18, 93.

53. In fact, studies in the United States (O'Malley, "Age-Based Rationing," 90) and internationally (Anthony P. Glascock, "By Any Other Name It Is Still Killing: A Comparison of the Treatment of the Elderly in America and Other Societies," in Jay Skolovsky, ed., *The Cultural Context of Aging: Worldwide Perspectives* [New York: Bergen and Garvey, 1990]: 53) reveal that where religious belief of a variety of forms is influential there is a reluctance to sup-

port age-based rationing and analogous practices that shorten the lives of elderly people.

54. These themes are developed and documented in Kilner, *Life on the Line,* 159ff.; Harris, *God and the Elderly.*

55. On the virtues of elderly persons, see William F. May, *The Patient's Ordeal* (Bloomington: Indiana University Press, 1991), 120–41. Post ("Justice for Elderly People," 131–32) and Stephen Sapp (*Full of Years: Aging and the Elderly in the Bible and Today* [Nashville: Abingdon Press, 1987], 133, 159) elaborate on the responsibility of older people to serve.

56. See also Post, "Justice for Elderly People," 126. Cf. Robert L. Barry, "Mandatory, Universal Age-Based Rationing of Scarce Medical Resources," in Barry and Bradley, eds., *Set No Limits,* 9; Thomasma, "From Ageism toward Autonomy," 146; Thomas H. Murray, "Meaning, Aging, and Public Policy," in Binstock and Post, eds., *Too Old for Health Care?* 178.

57. See Hauerwas, "Limits of Medicine," for more on story and community.

58. For much fuller, documented accounts of this perspective, see Kilner, *Life on the Line,* 54–57, 161–64, on life; and ibid., 97–103, on death. In these accounts, this view of life and death is distinguished from an un-Christian idolatry of life (i.e., vitalism) and paranoia about death (which leads to misguided attempts to prolong life at any cost). Cf. John Dunlop, "Death and Dying," in John F. Kilner, Arlene B. Miller, and Edmund D. Pellegrino, eds., *Dignity and Dying: A Christian Appraisal* (Grand Rapids: Eerdmans, 1996).

59. See George, "Life as an Evil," for an elaboration of the difference that views of life and death make for age-based allocation of health care.

60. See John F. Kilner, "Rationing and Health Care Reform," in John F. Kilner, Nigel M. De S. Cameron, and David L. Schiedermayer, eds., *Bioethics and the Future of Medicine: A Christian Appraisal* (Grand Rapids: Eerdmans, 1995), 290–301; Kilner, *Life on the Line,* 61–65; Stephen G. Post, "Justice for Elderly People in Jewish and Christian Thought," in Binstock and Post, eds., *Too Old for Health Care?* (Baltimore: Johns Hopkins University Press, 1991), 120; Catholic Health Association, Task Force on Long-Term Care Policy, *A Time to Be Old, A Time to Flourish: The Special Needs of the Elderly-at-Risk* (St. Louis: Catholic Health Association of the United States, 1988), 20.

61. For expanded figures and discussion, see Friedman, "Health Care's Changing Face," 37; Nancy S. Jecker, "Age-Based Rationing and Women," *Journal of the American Medical Association* 266 (Dec. 4, 1991): 3012–15; Nora K. Bell, "What Setting Limits May Mean: A Feminist Critique of Daniel Callahan's *Setting Limits,*" *Hypatia* 4 (Summer 1989): 176–77. Figures used here have been updated by the U.S. National Center for Health Statistics during July 1992. For a related analysis of class bias in age-based allocation, see Eliz-

abeth A. Binney and Carroll L. Estes, "The Paradox of Setting Limits," in Homer and Holstein, eds., *A Good Old Age?* 241. In his chapter in this book, Daniels admits that gender and class inequities might constitute valid reasons for rejecting age-based allocation.

62. Sapp, *Full of Years*, 122–25; Post, "Justice for Elderly People," 122–25.

63. See, for example, Mary M. Fulkerson, "Sexism as Original Sin: Developing a Theacentric Discourse," *Journal of the Academy of Religion* 59 (Winter 1991): 653–75.

64. This notion is developed in Karen Lebacqz, *Foundations of Justice* (Minneapolis: Augsburg Press, 1987), 151.

65. For example, see Norman Daniels, *Am I My Parents' Keeper? An Essay on Justice between the Young and the Old* (New York: Oxford University Press, 1988), 96; Daniels, *Just Health Care* (London: Cambridge University Press, 1985), 113; Margaret P. Battin, "Age Rationing and the Just Distribution of Health Care: Is There a Duty to Die?" *Ethics* 97 (Jan. 1987): 340. Daniels acknowledges that such age-based allocation would impose constraints on the liberty and welfare of elderly individuals that would in fact be experienced as unbearably harsh (*Just Health Care*, 99). For critiques that underscore the way that age-based allocation would magnify current injustices, see Barry, "Mandatory, Universal Age-Based Rationing," 5–11; Moody, *Ethics in an Aging Society*, 189–98; Post, "Justice for Elderly People," 127.

66. See Margret A. Somerville, "Justice across the Generations," *Social Science and Medicine* 29 (Feb. 1989): 393; Jecker and Pearlman, "Ethical Constraints of Rationing," 1073; Larry Churchill, "Should We Ration Health Care by Age?" *Journal of the American Geriatric Society* 36 (July 1988): 646–47; James F. Childress, "Artificial and Transplanted Organs," in James F. Childress et al., eds., *Biolaw*, vol. 1 (Frederick, Md.: University Publications of America, 1986), 318; Task Force on Organ Transplantation, *Organ Transplantation: Issues and Recommendations* (Rockville, Md.: U.S. Department of Health and Human Services, 1986), 90. On the importance of symbols (such as the provision of lifesaving health care) in shaping the way elderly persons are treated throughout society, see Maitland, *Aging*; Henry C. Simmons, "Countering Cultural Metaphors of Aging," *Journal of Religious Gerontology* 7:1–2 (1990): 160.

67. See especially Callahan, *Setting Limits*, 66–72, 170–73; Daniel Callahan, *What Kind of Life: The Limits of Medical Progress* (New York: Simon and Schuster, 1990), 151–54.

68. Callahan, *Setting Limits*, 66, 172. Accordingly, in the prologue to a collection of essays appraising Callahan's proposal, Nat Hentoff associates Callahan with what Hentoff characterizes as a basically utilitarian drift in health

care ("Prologue: The Indivisibility of Life," in Barry and Bradley, eds., *Set No Limits*, xi–xix).

69. Daniel Callahan, "Let the Elderly Choose," *New York Times*, July 12, 1993, A-13.

70. For example, Wetle, "Ethical Issues," 404; Post, "Justice for Elderly People," 129.

71. For more on this public strategy, see Cole, "Specter of Old Age," 93.

72. For more on aging as disease, failure, and evil, see Boyajian, "Sacrificing the Old," 325; Arluke and Peterson, "Accidental Medicalization," 277; Richard A. Kalish, "The New Ageism and the Failure Models: A Polemic," *The Gerontologist* 19 (Aug. 1979): 399.

73. On victim-blaming in general, see William Ryan, *Blaming the Victim* (New York: Random House, 1976). For analyses of the ways this orientation affects health care for elderly persons, see Kluge, "Calculus of Discrimination," 88; Cassel and Neugarten, "Goals of Medicine," 87; Murray, "Meaning, Aging," 178; Simmons, "Countering Cultural Metaphors," 155; Kane and Kane, *A Will and a Way*, 255.

74. See, for example, Glascock, "By Any Other Name," 45; Rachel Filinson and Stanley R. Ingman, *Elder Abuse: Practice and Policy* (New York: Human Sciences Press, 1989); Carl D. Chambers et al., eds., *Elderly: Victims and Deviants* (Athens: Ohio University Press, 1987); Karl A. Pillemer and Rosalie S. Wolf, *Elder Abuse: Conflict in the Family* (Westport, Conn.: Greenwood Press, 1986); Mary J. Quinn and Susan K. Tomita, *Elder Abuse and Neglect* (New York: Springer, 1986).

75. Claude Pepper, "Elder Abuse: The Problem That Still Persists," *Aging Network News*, Sept. 1986, 24–25; Glascock, "By Any Other Name," 45; Boyajian, "Sacrificing the Old," 321.

76. However, the example Battin favorably cites (in her essay in this volume) of the way that a country can give the term a specific definition and then maintain reassuring statistics on its implementation is less than reassuring. The Dutch definition, as Battin admits here, is so narrow that it does not even encompass all cases of directly ending a patient's life—much less morally related cases in which life-sustaining treatment is discontinued with the intention of ending a patient's life. So the resulting statistics concerning how often "euthanasia" is practiced—figures which she cites here—far from display the full extent to which the decisions are being made to end patients' lives. For more complete statistics, see Richard Fenigsen, "The Report of the Dutch Governmental Committee on Euthanasia," *Issues in Law and Medicine* 7 (Winter 1991): 339–44; cf. Carlos F. Gomez, *Regulating Death: The Case of the Netherlands* (New York: Free Press, 1991).

77. Gallup poll conducted for *Hospitals* magazine, reported in "New Poll Shows Americans Prefer Withdrawal in Irreversible Coma Cases," *Medical Ethics Advisor* 3 (May 1987): 64.

78. President's Commission for the Study of Ethical Problems in Medicine and Biomedical and Behavioral Research, *Deciding to Forgo Life-Sustaining Treatment* (Washington, D.C.: U.S. Government Printing Office, 1983).

79. For example, a study by Steven Neu and Carl M. Kjellstrand ("Stopping Long-Term Dialysis," *New England Journal of Medicine* 314 [Jan. 2, 1986]: 14–20) documents that by 1985, kidney dialysis was already being discontinued in one out of every eleven patients who had begun it. The authors suggest, moreover, that this figure may be understated. For an analysis of why the refusal of available treatment is underreported, see Alonzo L. Plough and Susanne Salem, "Social and Contextual Factors in the Analysis of Mortality in End-Stage Renal Disease Patients: Implications for Health Policy," *American Journal of Public Health* 72 (Nov. 1982): 1293–95.

80. Mervin D. Field, "California Poll: Strong Public Support for the Right to Die," *San Francisco Chronicle*, July 21, 1983, 12.

81. For a discussion of a 1986 Gallup poll and 1986 and 1988 Roper polls conducted in California, see Allan Parachini, "The California Humane and Dignified Death Initiative," *Hastings Center Report* 19 (Jan.–Feb. 1989): S11.

82. See Marcia Angell, "Euthanasia," *New England Journal of Medicine* 319 (Nov. 17, 1988): 1348–50; Roper Organization of New York City, *The Roper Poll on Attitudes toward Active Voluntary Euthanasia* (Los Angeles: National Hemlock Society, 1988). In addition, 49 percent of the people sampled in 1989 by the Chicago-based National Opinion Research Center agreed with the statement that people with incurable diseases have the right to end their lives ("View of Suicide as Right Disturbs Philosophers," *Bulletin of the Park Ridge Center* 5 [Sept. 1990]: 6–7). On a related issue, a 1990 *New York Times/CBS News* poll of 573 persons found that 53 percent agreed that physicians should be allowed to help patients take their own lives. A Roper poll that same year put the figure at 64 percent. On these and other polls, see Park Ridge Center for the Study of Health, Faith, and Ethics, *Active Euthanasia, Religion, and the Public Debate* (Chicago: Park Ridge Center, 1991), 31–32.

83. See, for example, the apparently real case reported in "It's Over, Debbie," *Journal of the American Medical Association* 259 (Jan. 8, 1988): 272, and the subsequent letters to the editor published in *JAMA* (259 [Apr. 8, 1988]: 2094–98; 260 [Aug. 12, 1988]: 787–89). For an actual case more recently reported, see Timothy E. Quill, "Death and Dignity: A Case of Individualized Decision-Making," *New England Journal of Medicine* 324 (Mar. 1991): 691–94, and subsequent letters to the editor (325 [Aug. 29, 1991]: 658–60). Re-

garding suicide devices, see "Suicide Device for Terminally Ill Raises Legal Ethical Concerns," *Lexington Herald Leader,* Oct. 29, 1989, E-6; Isabel Wilkerson, "Rage and Support for Doctor's Role in Suicide," *New York Times,* Oct. 25, 1991, A-1.

84. Sydney H. Wanzer et al., "The Physician's Responsibility toward Hopelessly Ill Patients: A Second Look," *New England Journal of Medicine* 320 (Mar. 30, 1989): 844–49; Daniel Q. Haney, "Panel Backs Doctor's Aiding in Suicides of Terminally Ill," *Lexington Herald Leader,* Mar. 30, 1989, 1, 5.

85. Parachini, "California Humane and Dignified Death." For a proposal by three prominent physicians to legalize physician-assisted suicide, see Timothy E. Quill et al., "Care of the Hopelessly Ill: Proposed Clinical Criteria for Physician-Assisted Suicide," *New England Journal of Medicine* 327 (Nov. 5, 1992): 1380–84.

86. See documentation and analysis in Melvin A. Kimble, "Religion: Friend or Foe of Aging?" *Second Opinion* 15 (Nov. 1990): 70–79; Moody, *Ethics in an Aging Society,* 73; Robert I. Simon, "Silent Suicide in the Elderly," *Bulletin of the American Academy of Psychiatry and Law* 17 (1989): 83–96; John L. McIntosh and Nancy J. Osgood, *Suicide and the Elderly* (Westport, Conn.: Greenwood Press, 1986).

87. See Glascock, "By Any Other Name."

88. Ibid., 55.

89. Robert N. Bellah et al., *Habits of the Heart* (Berkeley: University of California Press, 1985), broadly chart the individualism of U.S. culture. This theme is also highlighted by Estes and Binney in the present book. For discussions of the implications of this individualism (and consequent failure of community) for health care decisions and policy, see Moody, *Ethics in an Aging Society,* 4; Mark H. Waymack, "Old Age and the Rationing of Scarce Health Care Resources," in Jecker, ed., *Aging and Ethics,* 264; Larry Churchill, "Getting from 'I' to 'We,'" in Homer and Holstein, eds., *A Good Old Age?* 112; Hauerwas, "Limits of Medicine," 126.

90. For further reflection on the relationship between increasing government control and age-based resource allocation, see Barry, "Mandatory, Universal Age-Based Rationing," 8; Cassel, "Limits of Setting Limits," 197; Moody, *Ethics in an Aging Society,* 206.

Contributors

Margaret Pabst Battin is a professor of philosophy at the University of Utah. She is the author, editor, or coeditor of nine books, including *Should Medicine Be Rationed by Age?*, *Changing to National Health Care: The Ethical Issues*, and *The Least Worst Death: Essays in Bioethics on the End of Life*. She is currently working on issues of global population growth and reproductive rights.

Elizabeth A. Binney received her Ph.D. in sociology from the University of California at San Francisco and is a postdoctoral fellow in the Institute for Aging, Health, and Health Policy at Rutgers University. Her publications include "The Retreat of the State and Its Transfer of Responsibility," in the *International Journal of Health Services*.

Norman Daniels is chair of the Department of Philosophy at Tufts University. He has written extensively on allocation issues and is the author of *Am I My Parents' Keeper? An Essay on Justice between the Young and the Old* and *Just Health Care*.

Carroll L. Estes is a professor in and chair of the Department of Social and Behavioral Sciences and the director of the Institute for Health and Aging, all at the University of California at San Francisco. Among her many publications are "The Aging Enterprise Revisited," in *The Gerontologist*, and a coauthored chapter on "The Political Economy of Aging," in *Handbook of Aging and the Social Sciences* (4th ed.).

Nancy S. Jecker is an associate professor of medical history and ethics at the University of Washington. In addition to publishing numerous journal articles on rationing and the aged, she edited *Aging and Ethics: Philosophical Problems in Gerontology,* contributed to *The Encyclopedia of Gerontology,* and wrote chapters in the books *Geriatric Medicine* and *The Politics of Caring.*

Susan E. Kelly received her Ph.D. in medical sociology from the University of California at San Francisco and is a postdoctoral research fellow at the Stanford University Center for Biomedical Ethics. She currently chairs the research group on sociology of ethics, aging, and values in the American Sociology Association.

John F. Kilner is the director of the Center for Bioethics and Human Dignity in Chicago. The author of numerous articles in medical, public health, legal, religious, and ethics journals, his most recent books are *Life on the Line: Ethics, Aging, Ending Patients' Lives, and Allocating Vital Resources* and *Who Lives? Who Dies?—Ethical Criteria in Patient Selection.*

Paul T. Menzel is a professor of philosophy and provost at Pacific Lutheran University. He is the author of *Strong Medicine: The Ethical Rationing of Health Care* and *Medical Costs, Moral Choices: A Philosophy of Health Care Economics in America,* as well as articles in ethics, social philosophy, and health policy.

James W. Walters, professor of ethical studies at Loma Linda University, directed the Ethics and Aging Project in Southern California that made this anthology possible. His five books include *Facing Limits: Ethics and Health Care for the Elderly.* He is currently working on definitions of death and morally valuable life in light of brain function.

Index